Yoga for your Brain

Tim Sole

&

Rod Marshall

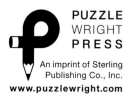

PUZZLE
WRIGHT
PRESS

An imprint of Sterling
Publishing Co., Inc.

www.puzzlewright.com

Dedication

Because they were

$$\begin{array}{r} 2 \text{ good} \\ 2 \text{ us} \\ 2 \text{ be} \\ \underline{4} \text{ got} \\ 10 \end{array}$$

this book is dedicated to our families, who have accepted with remarkable patience our fascination with puzzles. To Liz, Heather, and Lynsey Marshall, and Judy, David, Zoe, and Catherine Sole. We hope you will be pleased with the prospect of seeing more of us again, and we hope you enjoy this book.

Puzzlewright Press and the distinctive Puzzlewright Press logo are trademarks of Sterling Publishing Co., Inc.

2   4   6   8   10   9   7   5   3   1

Puzzles in this book appeared previously in *Nearly Impossible Brain Bafflers*, *You'd Better Be Really Smart Brain Bafflers*, and *Almost Impossible Brain Bafflers*, © 1998, 2003, and 2006
by Tim Sole and Rod Marshall
Published by Sterling Publishing Co., Inc.
387 Park Avenue South, New York, NY 10016
© 2009 by Sterling Publishing Co., Inc.
Distributed in Canada by Sterling Publishing
C/o Canadian Manda Group, 165 Dufferin Street
Toronto, Ontario, Canada M6K 3H6
Distributed in the United Kingdom by GMC Distribution Services
Castle Place, 166 High Street, Lewes, East Sussex, England BN7 1XU
Distributed in Australia by Capricorn Link (Australia) Pty. Ltd.
P.O. Box 704, Windsor, NSW 2756, Australia

Sterling ISBN 978-1-4027-6707-4

For information about custom editions, special sales, premium and corporate purchases, please contact Sterling Special Sales Department at 800-805-5489 or specialsales@sterlingpublishing.com.

Contents

Acknowledgments

Our thanks are due to many people, without whose help this book would not have been possible. To name but a few:

Our respective wives, Judy Sole and Liz Marshall, without whose support this book would never have happened.

The London Staple Inn Actuarial Society, which publishes *The Actuary* and which published its predecessor, *Fiasco*. Many of the puzzles in this book have been published in one of these magazines.

Roger Gilbert, former puzzle editor for the magazine *Actuary Australia*, and creator of some very fine puzzles.

The editors of *The Actuary*, *Fiasco*, and *Actuary Australia* for their support and encouragement to us as puzzle editors.

Those listed below (and we apologize if we have overlooked anyone) for creating, assisting with, or suggesting puzzles that we have used:

14–Heather Marshall, 30–David Walters, 33–Terry Wills, 55–Roger Gilbert, 60–L.J. Gray, 61–Steven Haberman, 62–K.J. Fagg, 65–Danny Roth, 69–Terry Wills, 72–John Sant, 80–Maurice Steinhart, 83–Paul McHugh, 101–David Twigger, 127–David Wharton, 150–H.E. Dudeney, 175–David Sole, 188–Maurice Steinhart, 202–Edward Johnston, 222–Chris Munro, 225–Roger Gilbert, 231–Chris Cole, 237–Maurice Steinhart, 240–Charles G. Groeschell, 247–Alan Wood, 255–Hugh Norman, 256–David Sole, 257–Alan Wilson, John Gemmell, Tom Grimes, 258–Terry Wills, Francis Heaney, 259–D.P. Laurie, 260–Dennis Lister, 266–Tim Lund, 292–Frank Guaschi, 306–Pat O'Keefe,

309–David Kerr, 311–Alan Wilson, 322–Roger Gilbert and P.C. Wickens, 336–Alexander T. Brooks, 339–David Sole, 340–Chris Cole, 360–Roger Gilbert, 365–Tad Dunne, 367–Terry Wills, 369–Phil Watson and Kevin Kelly, 372–H.E. Dudeney, 382–Neil Parrack, 406–Henry Garfath, 408–Roger Gilbert, 417–Roger Gilbert, 418–Roger Gilbert.

—Tim Sole and Rod Marshall

PUZZLES

1. What word, expression, or name is depicted below?

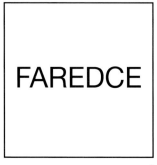

FAREDCE

Answer, page 181

2. Find a ten-digit number containing each digit once, so that the number formed by the first n digits is divisible by n for each value of n between 1 and 10.

Answer, page 175

3. When the examination results were published, one college found that all 32 of its students were successful in at least one of the three exams that each of them had taken. Of the students who did not pass Exam One, the number who passed Exam Two was exactly half of the number who passed Exam Three. The number who passed only Exam One was the same as the number who passed only one of the other two exams, and three more than the number who passed Exam One and at least one of the other two exams.

How many students passed more than one exam?

Answer, page 177

4. If 89 players enter a single elimination tennis tournament, how many matches would it take to decide the winner, excluding byes?

Answer, page 203

5. Using exactly two 2's and any of the standard mathematical symbols, write down an expression whose value is five.

Answer, page 177

6. What word, expression, or name is depicted below?

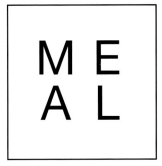

Answer, page 200

7. This puzzle was devised by Dr. Karl Fabel and published in 1949 in "T.R.D.'s Diamond Jubilee" issue of the *Fairy Chess Review*.

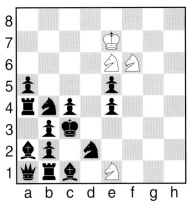

White to play and mate in sixty.

Answer, page 180

8. What word, expression, or name is depicted below?

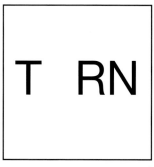

Answer, page 179

9. Find a ten-digit number whose first digit is the number of ones in the number, whose second digit is the number of twos in the number, whose third digit is the number of threes in the number, and so on up to the tenth digit, which is the number of zeros in the number.

Answer, page 189

10. Without using a calculator, guess which is bigger: e^π or π^e?

Answer, page 202

11. A selection of eight cards is dealt with every second card being returned to the bottom of the pack. Thus the top card goes to the table, card two goes to the bottom of the pack, card three goes to the table, card four to the bottom of the pack, and so on. This procedure continues until all the cards are dealt.

The order in which the cards appear on the table is:

A K A K A K A K

How were the cards originally stacked?

Answer, page 177

12. Gambler A chooses a series of three possible outcomes from successive throws of a die, depending simply on whether the number thrown each time is odd (O) or even (E). Gambler B then chooses a different series of three successive possible outcomes. The die is then thrown as often as necessary until either gambler's chosen series of outcomes occurs.

For example, Gambler A might choose the series EOE and B might choose OEE. If successive throws gave, say, EEOOEOE, then A would win the game after the seventh throw. Had the sixth throw been E rather than O, then B would have won.

A has chosen the series EEE and B, who was thinking of choosing OEE, changes his mind to OOO. Has B reduced his chance of winning the game or is it still the same?

Answer, page 203

13. What word, expression, or name is depicted below?

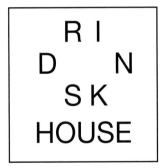

Answer, page 188

14. Find three different two-digit primes where the average of any two is a prime, and the average of all three is a prime.

Answer, page 193

15. Each letter in the sum below represents a different digit. Can you crack the code and discover the uncoded sum?

```
    T   W   E   L   V   E
    T   W   E   L   V   E
    T   W   E   L   V   E
    T   W   E   L   V   E
    T   W   E   L   V   E
+   T   H   I   R   T   Y
─────────────────────────
    N   I   N   E   T   Y
```

Answer, page 198

16. A spider is in a rectangular warehouse measuring $40 \times 10 \times 10$ meters. The spider is on the 10-by-10-meter wall, 5 meters from the sides and 1 meter above the ground. The proverbial fly is on the opposite wall 5 meters from the sides and 1 meter below the ceiling. What is the shortest route for the spider to walk to the fly?

Answer, page 204

17. What word, expression, or name is depicted below?

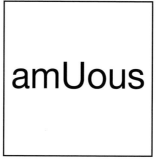

Answer, page 183

18. In a game of table tennis, 24 of the 37 points played were won by the player serving, and Smith beat Jones 21-16. Remembering in table tennis that service alternates every five points, who served first?

Answer, page 175

19. This chess puzzle by C.S. Kipping was published in the *Manchester City News* in 1911.

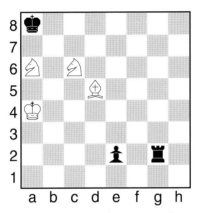

White to play and mate in three.

Answer, page 176

20. What word, expression, or name is depicted below?

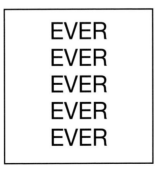

EVER
EVER
EVER
EVER
EVER

Answer, page 183

21. In the three envelopes shown, the statements on one of the three are both true, the statements on another are both false, and the remaining envelope has one statement that is true and one that is false.

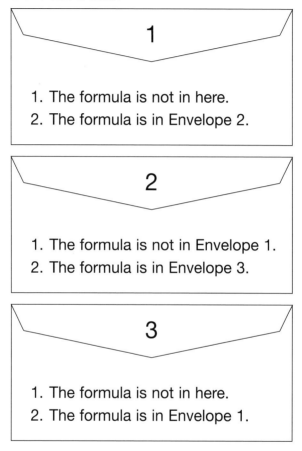

1

1. The formula is not in here.
2. The formula is in Envelope 2.

2

1. The formula is not in Envelope 1.
2. The formula is in Envelope 3.

3

1. The formula is not in here.
2. The formula is in Envelope 1.

Which envelope contains the formula?

Answer, page 175

22. How can eleven matches make nine, nine matches make ten, and ten matches make five?

Answer, page 201

23. Caesar and Brutus are playing a game in which each says the next number from a well-known sequence. The first 20 terms of the sequence are given below:

1 2 3 2 1 2 3 4 2 1 2 3 4 3 2 3 4 5 3 2

The fortieth term is 2. If Caesar began the game, who will be the first to say 10?

Answer, page 177

24. This (okay, somewhat misshapen) Valentine heart consists of one large semicircle beneath two smaller semicircles. The arrow passes right through the point at which the two smaller semicircles meet.

Which part of the heart's perimeter is the longer: that lying above the line of the arrow, or that lying below?

Answer, page 187

25. What word, expression, or name is depicted below?

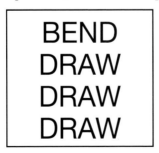

BEND
DRAW
DRAW
DRAW

Answer, page 192

26. This week's chart of the top 40 pop songs has just been published. The song that was at number 35 in last week's chart has dropped out, and there is a new entry at number 32. There are also five non-movers, at positions 1, 23, 29, 31, and 37. Of the other 34 songs in the new chart, 18 have moved up and 16 down, but in every instance the number of positions moved, whether up or down, was a factor (greater than one, but possibly equal to the number itself) of the song's position in last week's chart.

The titles of last week's top 40 are shown below. Complete this week's chart.

Last week		This week	Last week		This week
Atomic	1	Atomic	Valentine	21	
Blockbuster	2		What	22	
Classic	3		Xanadu	23	Xanadu
Dizzy	4		YMCA	24	
Emma	5		Zabadak!	25	
Footloose	6		Autumn Almanac	26	
Gaye	7		Angie Baby	27	
Hello	8		Another Day	28	
Intuition	9		Angel Eyes	29	Angel Eyes
Jesamine	10		Angel Fingers	30	
Kayleigh	11		Amateur Hour	31	Amateur Hour
Lamplight	12		Angela Jones	32	New entry
Mickey	13		Ain't Nobody	33	
Night	14		American Pie	34	
Obsession	15		Ant Rap	35	
Perfect	16		Alphabet Street	36	
Question	17		Alternate Title	37	Alternate Title
Reward	18		As Usual	38	
Sandy	19		Adoration Waltz	39	
True	20		Always Yours	40	

Answer, page 199

27. What word, expression, or name is depicted below?

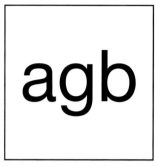

Answer, page 175

28. The following was originally a list of five-letter words, but in each case two consecutive letters (though never the first two) have been removed. The 26 missing letters are all different. What was the original list?

A	N	T
A	S	S
B	A	Y
C	O	Y
D	I	M
E	E	L
F	A	R
M	A	R
P	I	E
S	E	E
T	I	E
T	O	P
W	I	N

Answer, page 174

29. There is one in a minute and two in a moment, but only one in a million years. What are we talking about?

Answer, page 205

30. Find nine different integers from 1 to 20 inclusive such that no combination of any three of the nine integers form an arithmetic progression. For example, if two of the integers chosen were 7 and 13, then that would preclude 1, 10, and 19 from being included.

Answer, page 179

31. This puzzle was composed by Hans August and Dr. Karl Fabel, and was published in 1949 in *Romana de Sah*.

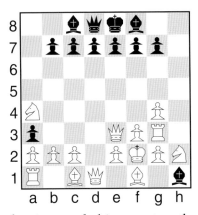

White has just made his seventeenth move.
What was Black's ninth move, and what
were the moves that followed it?

Answer, page 202

32. Two travelers set out at the same time to travel opposite ways round a circular railway. Trains start each way on the hour, 15 minutes past, half past, and 45 minutes past. Clockwise trains take two hours for the journey, counterclockwise trains take three hours. Including trains seen at the starting point and the ones they are traveling on, how many trains did each traveler see on his journey?

Answer, page 193

33. The Roman numerals still in use are I = 1, V = 5, X = 10, L = 50, C = 100, D = 500, and M = 1000. Examples of four Roman numbers are VIII = 8, LXXVI = 76, CXXXVI = 136, and MDCCCLXII = 1862.

Today, the Roman numbers IIII, VIIII, and DCCCC are usually abbreviated as IV, IX, and CM, respectively, a numeral to the left of a higher numeral denoting subtraction. Where there is an opportunity, these abbreviations are used in this cross-number, together with CD for CCCC, XC for LXXXX, and XL for XXXX. Thus 1904 would be written as MCMIV and 49 as XLIX. Note that the logical extension of this method of abbreviation, such as IL for 49, for example, was never fully developed and so is not used here. All that is used, where there is an opportunity, are the six usual abbreviations already mentioned.

In the grid below all answers are Roman numerals and, when converted to Arabic (normal) numbers, are palindromes (none starting with zero) of two digits or more. One number occurs twice, the rest are all different.

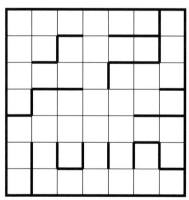

Answer, page 198

34. We place in a box 13 white marbles and 15 black. We also have 28 black marbles outside the box.

We remove two marbles from the box. If they have a different color, we put the white one back in the box. If they have the same color, we put a black marble in the box. We continue doing this until only one marble is left in the box. What is its color?

Answer, page 186

35. What word, expression, or name is depicted below?

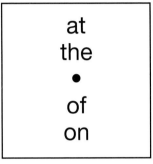

Answer, page 182

36. A drawer contains a number of red and blue socks. If I pull two out at random, then the chance of them being a red pair is a half and the chance of them being a blue pair is a twelfth. How many socks are in the drawer?

Answer, page 193

37. A long time ago, you could buy eight hens for a dollar or one sheep for a dollar, and cows were ten dollars each. A farmer buying animals of each type bought a hundred animals for a hundred dollars. What animals did he buy?

Answer, page 195

38. What word, expression, or name is depicted below?

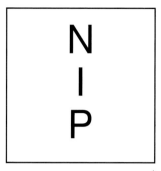

Answer, page 183

39. Are 1997 nickels worth more than 1992 nickels?

Answer, page 185

40. Insert the missing letter:

J ? M A M J J A

Answer, page 184

41. In a league of four soccer teams, each team played the other three teams. Two points were awarded for a win and one point for a tie. After all six games were played, a final league table was prepared, as shown below:

Team	Won	Tied	Lost	Goals for	Goals against	Points
A	3	0	0	6	1	6
B	1	1	1	2	4	3
C	1	0	2	2	2	2
D	0	1	2	2	5	1

What was the score in each of the six games?

Answer, page 190

42. Lynsey is a biology student. Her project for this term is measuring the effect of an increase in vitamin C in the diet of 25 laboratory mice. Each mouse will have a different diet supplement of between 1 to 50 units. Fractions of a unit are not possible.

Although the university pays for the mice's food, Lynsey has to buy the vitamin C supplement herself. The first consideration in designing this experiment was therefore to minimize the total number of supplements.

The second consideration was that no mouse should have an exact multiple of another mouse's supplement. Thus, if one mouse was on a supplement of 14 units, then this would preclude supplements of 1, 2, 7, 28, and 42 units.

What supplements should Lynsey use?

Answer, page 181

43. Find two ten-digit numbers, each containing the digits from 0 to 9 once and once only, with the property that successive pairs of digits, from left to right, are divisible in turn by 2, 3, 4, 5, 6, 7, 8, 9, and 10.

Answer, page 184

44. What word, expression, or name is depicted below?

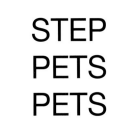

Answer, page 188

45. What are the numbers in the tenth line of the following pyramid?

1

1 1

2 1

1 2 1 1

1 1 1 2 2 1

3 1 2 2 1 1

1 3 1 1 2 2 2 1

1 1 1 3 2 1 3 2 1 1

3 1 1 3 1 2 1 1 1 1 3 1 2 2 1

Answer, page 183

46. What word, expression, or name is depicted below?

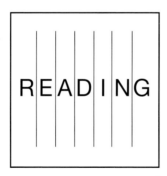

Answer, page 188

47. What digit does each letter represent in the multiplication below, given that no two letters stand for the same digit?

LAGER

× 4

REGAL

Answer, page 186

48. The order of the clues has been muddled up, but 21-Across is correct.

Answer, page 196

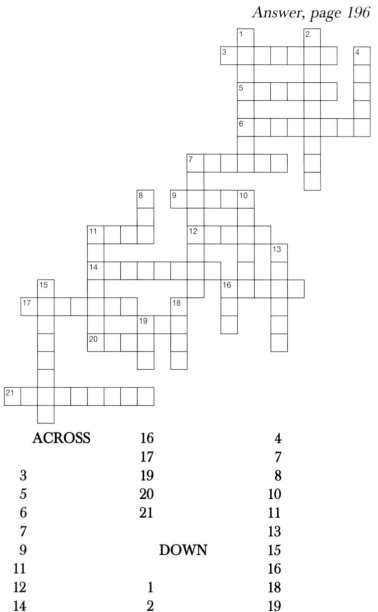

ACROSS	16	4
	17	7
3	19	8
5	20	10
6	21	11
7		13
9		15
11	DOWN	16
12		18
14	1	19
	2	

49. What word, expression, or name is depicted below?

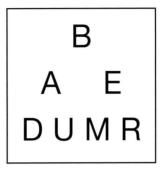

Answer, page 194

50. Letters other than "x" each represent a different digit. An "x," however, may represent any digit. There is no remainder. Find which digits the letters and each "x" stand for:

```
                O  N  E
    T  R  Y ) T  H  I  S  x
             x  x  x
                x  x  x
                x  x  x
                x  x  x  x
                x  x  x  x
```

Answer, page 205

51. The number 6 has factors (not counting itself) of 1, 2, and 3, which add up to 6. The number 28 has the same property, since its factors, 1, 2, 4, 7, and 14, add up to 28. What four-digit number has this property?

Answer, page 185

52. Between noon and midnight, but not counting these times, how often will the minute hand and hour hand of a clock overlap?

Answer, page 181

53. What word, expression, or name is depicted below?

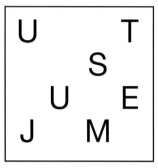

Answer, page 203

54. A set of building blocks contains a number of wooden cubes. The six faces of each cube are painted, each with a single color, in such a way that no two adjacent faces have the same color. Given that only five different colors have been used and that no two of the blocks are identical in their colorings, what is the maximum number of blocks there can be in the set?

Answer, page 176

55. The Bowls Club has fewer than 100 members. To the nearest whole number, 28% of the members are former committee members, 29% are current committee members, and 42% have never been on the committee. Again to the nearest whole number, 35% of the former committee members are women. What is the total membership of the club?

Answer, page 178

56. The pars for a nine-hole golf course designed by a mathematician are:

3 3 5 4 4 3 5 5 4

On which very well-known series (as well-known as one, two, three, etc.) are the pars based?

Answer, page 183

57. This may seem self-contradictory, but find three integers in arithmetic progression (that is, with equal differences, such as 230, 236, and 242) whose product is prime.

Answer, page 198

58. What is the next term in this series?:

1248 1632 6412 8256

Answer, page 181

59. What word, expression, or name is depicted below?

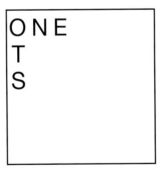

Answer, page 179

60. The ages of Old and Young total 48. Old is twice as old as Young was when Old was half as old as Young will be when Young is three times as old as Old was when Old was three times as old as Young. How old is Old?

Answer, page 188

61. Consider a five-by-five version of a chessboard with one player having five queens and the other player three queens. There are no other pieces. Can you place the queens on the board so that neither player's queens can capture one of his or her opponent's queens?

Answer, page 195

62.

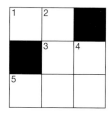

ACROSS
1 Starting piece between 3 and 4
3 2-Down minus a perfect square
5 Three!

DOWN
2 A perfect square
4 1.5 times 5-Across (or two-thirds of 5-Across)

Answer, page 175

63. What word, expression, or name is depicted below?

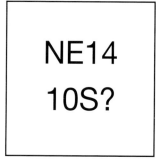

Answer, page 186

64. A full set of dominoes (0-0 to 6-6) has been laid out in a rectangular array. The numbers in the diagram represent the spots on the dominoes, and the puzzle is to identify the position of each domino within the pattern.

```
1 2 6 1 6 3 4 5
3 3 6 4 3 2 5 4
3 0 6 0 3 1 2 2
0 5 5 4 6 5 0 2
0 2 5 1 5 0 0 1
6 4 3 4 4 1 1 1
2 2 6 4 5 0 3 6
```

Answer, page 198

65. At the end of the soccer season, every player had scored a prime number of goals and the average for the eleven players was also a prime number. No player's tally was the same as anyone else's, and neither was it the same as the average.

Given that nobody had scored more than 45 goals, how many goals did each player score?

Answer, page 186

66. What word, expression, or name is depicted below?

timing

tim   ing

Answer, page 184

67. Allwyn, Aitkins, and Arthur are to fight a three-way duel. The order in which they shoot will be determined by lot and they will continue to shoot until two are dead. Allwyn never misses, Aitkins is 80% accurate, and Arthur, the cleverest of the three, hits his target just half of the time. Who has the best chance of surviving?

Answer, page 191

68. What word, expression, or name is depicted below?

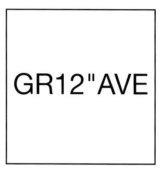

Answer, page 193

69. Can you subdivide a square measuring eleven by eleven into five rectangles such that the five lengths and five widths of the rectangles are all different and integral? There are two solutions.

Answer, page 195

70. What are the missing numbers?

31   62   __   25   56   __   19

Answer, page 196

71. Find three different positive integers whose factorials are each one less than a perfect square, and whose factorials sum to a perfect square.

Answer, page 185

72. I recently overheard a conversation that went roughly as follows:

Bob: "Here's a problem that might interest you. On my bus this morning there were only three other passengers, all of whom I knew. We discovered that the product of their ages was 2,450, and that the sum was exactly twice your age. How old are they?"

Jim: "Hang on. You haven't given me enough info."

Bob: "Oh, sorry. I forgot to mention that one of the passengers on the bus was someone older than me, and I am—"

Jim: "I know how old you are. And I now know the passengers' ages, too."

How old are Jim, Bob, and each of the three other passengers?

Answer, page 191

73. This puzzle is based on a theme by W.A. Shinkman, and the mate-in-three was first solved by Sam Loyd. The puzzle below was published in the *Leeds Mercury Supplement* in 1895.

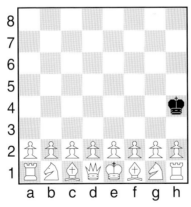

White to play and mate in three.

Answer, page 200

74. Construct a game that will leave the position shown for Puzzle 73 after Black's sixteenth move.

Answer, page 201

75. In a game of poker, one of the hands of five cards had the following features:
• There was no card above a 10 (an ace is above a 10 in poker).
• No two cards were of the same value.
• All four suits were represented.
• The total values of the odd and even cards were equal.
• No three cards were in sequence.
• The black cards totaled 10 in value.
• The hearts totaled 14.
• The lowest card was a spade.
  What was the hand?

Answer, page 175

76. What word, expression, or name is depicted below?

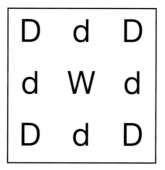

Answer, page 200

77. "Bookkeeper" has three consecutive double letters. What common two-word phrase, if you remove the space, also has three consecutive double letters?

Answer, page 186

78. What word, expression, or name is depicted below?

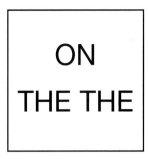

Answer, page 177

79. Divide the following figure into four identical parts, with each part made up of whole squares only. Each of the four parts should also contain one O and one X, but not necessarily in the same relative positions.

O			X		
			X		
		O			
	X		X		
			O	O	

Answer, page 193

80. Using each of the numbers 1, 5, 6, and 7 once and once only, parentheses as required, and any combination and any number of the following symbols:

$$+ \ - \ \times \ /$$

find an expression that equals 21.

Answer, page 194

81. P and Q are integers that between them contain each of the digits from 0 to 9 once and once only. What is the maximum value of P × Q?

Answer, page 181

82. What word, expression, or name is depicted below?

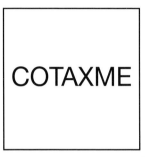

Answer, page 184

83. A total of five triangles can be seen in the diagram on the left.

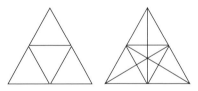

How many triangles can be found in the diagram on the right?

Answer, page 188

84. Using just four sixes, parentheses where necessary, and the following seven symbols as needed:

$$+ \quad - \quad \times \quad / \quad . \quad ! \quad \sqrt{}$$

find an expression for 29.

Answer, page 192

85. What word, expression, or name is depicted below?

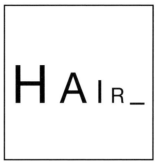

Answer, page 191

86. In this long division, each "x" represents a digit. Find which digits each "x" stands for:

```
                  x   x . x   x   x
  x   x  )   x   x   x   x
              x   x
              x   x   x
              x   x
                  x   x
                  x   x
                  x   x   x
                  x   x   x
                      x   x
                      x   x
```

Answer, page 192

87. What are the two missing numbers in the series below?
    _ _ 3 3 7 7 2 3 6 5

Answer, page 186

88. Five soccer teams, United, County, Rovers, Albion, and Thistle, took part in a league tournament. Their colors were white, yellow, green, red, and blue, though not necessarily in that order. No teams were tied in the standings at the end of the tournament. From the following information, determine for each team its captain, colors, and position in which it finished in the league.

• Rovers did not win the league, but finished higher than fourth.

• Neither Albion nor the team in green finished in the top three.

• Evans captained the team in yellow.

• Cooke's team finished ahead of County, which was captained by Dixon

• Allen's team finished second and Boyle's team finished last.

• The team in white finished lower than both United and the team in blue, but above Evans's team.

• Albion was not the green team and United was not the blue team.

Answer, page 174

89. What word, expression, or name is depicted below?

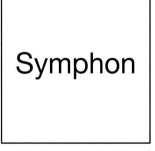

Answer, page 195

90. Arrange the digits from 1 to 9 in a 3 × 3 array in such a way that the sum of a number's immediate neighbors (including diagonals) is a multiple of that number.

9	5	1
6	7	2
4	3	8

The example shows an unsatisfactory attempt. The three numbers bordering 9 add to 18, which is a multiple of 9 as required, and the numbers bordering 1, 2, 3, 4, and 5 also meet the condition specified. The numbers bordering 6, 7, and 8, however, do not meet the required condition.

Answer, page 186

91. What word, expression, or name is depicted below?

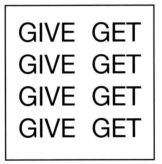

Answer, page 174

92. What is the minimum difference between two integers that between them contain each digit once?

Answer, page 175

93. This position was created by F. Amelung and published in *Düna Zeitung* in 1897. It is a puzzle that has since defeated many good chess players, and one cannot but wonder whether it has ever occurred naturally in a real game. If it did, and you were White and about to play, how could you force mate in two?

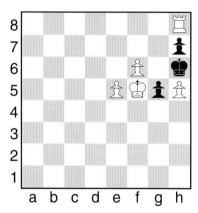

White to play and mate in two.

Answer, page 191

94. Arrange the digits from one to nine in a 3×3 square in such a way that each of the three-digit numbers reading across, and the three-digit number on the diagonal from top left to bottom right, are all perfect squares.

Answer, page 200

95. The digital root of a number is obtained by summing its digits and then repeating this process until the answer is a single digit. For example, the digital root of 8777 is 2.

Noting that any number divisible by nine has a digital root of nine, what is the digital root of $\left(9^{6130} + 2\right)^{4875}$?

Answer, page 203

96. If six equilateral triangles each of unit area are joined edge-to-edge, twelve different shapes each of six units in area can be constructed as shown below:

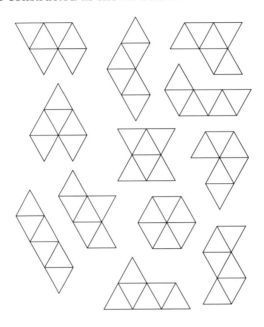

Show that it is impossible to form any six of these shapes into a six-by-six-by-six equilateral triangle of 36 units in area.

Answer, page 178

97. Which of the following poker hands is stronger?

A♣	A♦	A♥	K♣	K♥

or

A♣	A♥	K♣	K♦	K♠

Think about it!

Answer, page 194

98. Continue the sequence:

202 122 232 425 262 728 ? ?

Answer, page 177

99. What word, expression, or name is depicted below?

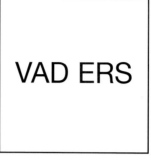

Answer, page 201

100. The third and fourth powers of this integer contain between them exactly one of each digit. What is the integer?

Answer, page 192

101. Complete the eight words using each letter of the alphabet once and once only.

```
_ A _ E R I _ _
_ U _ _ _ E
_ I _ _ E
_ _ L _ E R
_ I _ _
_ _ A P
B R _ _ _ N
_ O L _ _ A _
```

Answer, page 188

102.
*Is the tenth root of ten
A little bit more
Than the root of the square
Of the sixth root of four?*

Answer, page 174

103. This cross-number uses Roman numbers only and yes, every clue is the same! If you are struggling to remember what the Roman numerals are and how they are used, a description is given in Puzzle 33.

ACROSS

1 A perfect square
7 A perfect square
8 A perfect square
9 A perfect square
10 A perfect square
13 A perfect square
14 A perfect square
17 A perfect square
19 A perfect square
20 A perfect square

DOWN

1 A perfect square
2 A perfect square
3 A perfect square
4 A perfect square
5 A perfect square
6 A perfect square
7 A perfect square
11 A perfect square
12 A perfect square
15 A perfect square
16 A perfect square
18 A perfect square
19 A perfect square

Answer, page 183

104. What word, expression, or name is depicted below?

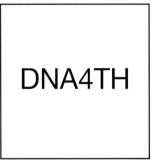

DNA4TH

Answer, page 181

105. A horizontal line from the top of the inside edge of a bicycle tire to the two outside edges of the tire measures 24 centimeters as shown in the side view below:

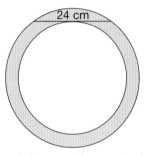

24 cm

What is the area of the bicycle tire visible from this view?
Answer, page 185

106. In the following line, cross out six letters so that the remaining letters, without altering their sequence, will spell a familiar English word.

B S A I N X L E A T N T E A R S

Answer, page 175

107. What word, expression, or name is depicted below?

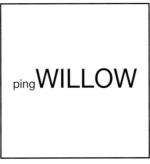

Answer, page 188

108. What is the smallest integer that can be expressed as the sum of two squares in three different ways? The answer is less than 500.

Answer, page 185

109. Two right triangles share the same hypotenuse AB. The shorter sides of the first triangle are 13 and 18 units; the shorter sides of the second are 7 and 20 units.

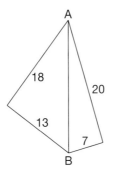

Clearly we are not measuring in base 10. What base is being used, and how long is the hypotenuse?

Answer, page 197

110. A ball with a diameter of 40 centimeters is lying on the ground, tight against a wall:

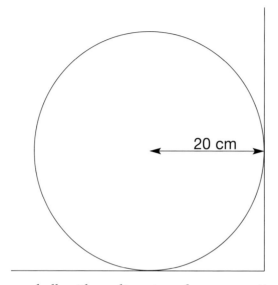

20 cm

Can a ball with a diameter of seven centimeters pass through the gap between the ball, ground, and wall?

Answer, page 182

111. What word, expression, or name is depicted below?

1 D   5 U
2 R   6 L
3 A   7 A
4 C

Answer, page 183

112. What word, expression, or name is depicted below?

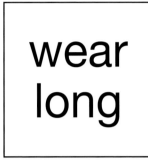

Answer, page 177

113. This puzzle by Sam Loyd was published in the *Holyoke Transcript* in 1876.

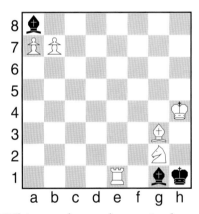

White to play and mate in three.

Answer, page 189

114. "Strength" is an eight-letter word with only one vowel. What's an eight-letter word with five vowels in a row?

Answer, page 194

115. The array of blocks shown below spells the word "PUZZLE." Could we be looking at six different views of the same block, or is one or more of the views inconsistent with the others?

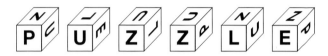

Answer, page 193

116. What word, expression, or name is depicted below?

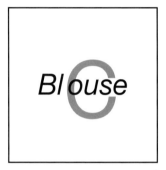

Answer, page 199

117. Using the digits one to nine in ascending order and no more than three standard arithmetical signs, find an expression that equals 100. An example that uses six standard arithmetical signs is shown below:

$$1 + (2 \times 3) - 4 + (56 \div 7) + 89 = 100$$

Answer, page 195

118. If the integers that contain each digit once were arranged in ascending order, which would be the millionth? (Numbers can't start with 0.)

Answer, page 188

119. A Christmas decoration comprises a symmetrical four-pointed star supported by three threads. The decoration hangs in the center of a small circular window:

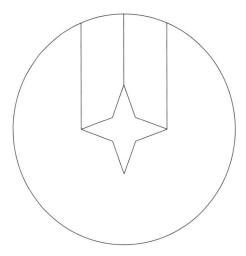

The central thread is 4 centimeters long, and the outer two are each 6 centimeters long. What is the width of the star?

Answer, page 197

120. What word, expression, or name is depicted below?

79 S 34 A 92

F 185 E 376

7 T 27 Y 12

Answer, page 181

121. Without using a calculator, determine which is greater: $3^{1/8} \times 3^{1/5}$ or $3 \times \sqrt[3]{37}$?

Answer, page 182

122. In the expression below, do the three letters represent three different digits?

$$(\textbf{ANNE})_{\text{base 8}} - (\textbf{ANNE})_{\text{base 5}} = (\textbf{ANNE})_{\text{base 7}}$$

Answer, page 184

123. Eric the Halibut is swimming to the right. Move three sticks (and his eye, smile, and bubbles) so that he is swimming to the left.

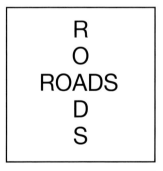

Answer, page 199

124. What word, expression, or name is depicted below?

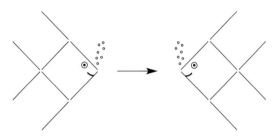

Answer, page 200

125. Losers' Chess is a fun game that often turns in a surprise result. To play it, ignore checks and checkmates, for the object is either to lose all of one's men, king included, or be stalemated (unable to play a move). Players must capture an opponent's man if they can, but where there is a choice, can choose which. All other rules are the same as for ordinary chess.

Puzzles in Losers' Chess are rare, and ones with an unusual twist like the one below even rarer. This one, by T.R. Dawson, was first published in 1925 in *Das Wochenschach*. In the first analysis it looks like Black can force White to stalemate him, but White, who is playing up the board, can play and win by forcing Black to cause the stalemate. How?

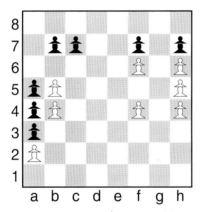

White to play and win (Losers' Chess rules).

Answer, page 185

126. A ladder 5 meters long leans against a wall. A box measuring 1 × 1 × 1 meters just fits in the gap. If the base of the ladder is nearer to the wall than the top of the ladder is to the ground, how far is the base of the ladder from the wall?

Answer, page 179

127. No answer begins with a zero.

ACROSS

1 See 3-Down
3 A multiple of 3
8 3 × 17-Down
9 2 × 15-Down
10 See 14-Down
11 See 6-Down
13 2 × 4-Down
16 Not 3-Down
18 See 5-Down
20 2 × 2-Down
21 Not 6-Down
22 See 1-Down
23 Same as 20-Down

DOWN

1 2 × 22-Across
2 See 20-Across
3 2 × 1-Across
4 See 13-Across
5 2 × 18-Across
6 3 × 11-Across
7 Same as 23-Across
12 2 × 3-Across
14 2 × 10-Across + 4
15 See 9-Across
17 See 8-Across
19 Square of 23-Across
20 See 23-Across

Answer, page 192

128. What number, when spelled out, has no repeated letters and has each of the vowels (not including **Y**) once?

Answer, page 194

129. What word, expression, or name is depicted below?

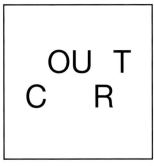

Answer, page 186

130. Shown below are six numbered pool balls arranged in a triangular pattern such that each number in the pattern is equal to the difference between the two numbers above:

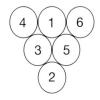

Find a similar triangular pattern for fifteen pool balls numbered 1 to 15.

Answer, page 200

131. What is the next term in this series?

100 121 144 202 244 400 ...

Answer, page 181

132. What are the next two letters in the following series and why?

W A T N T L I T F S _ _

Answer, page 176

133. The diagram shows a regular pentagram:

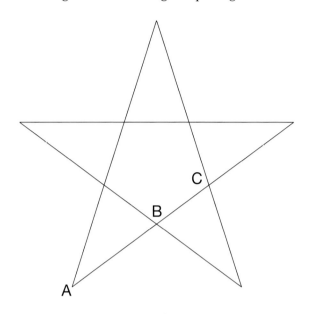

What is the ratio of AB to BC?

Answer, page 190

134.
If B is two A,
C three A plus B,
And A is "eleven eleven,"
Is B to the C
Plus C to the B
Divisible by seven?

"Eleven eleven,"
So you won't be confused,
Has nothing to do with odd bases.
It's simply ten thou
That's multiplied by
One ninth to four decimal places.

Answer, page 203

135. Reconstruct the following multiplication, using the digits 2, 3, 5, and 7 only.

```
        x   x   x
            x   x
    ─────────────────
    x   x   x   x
x   x   x   x
─────────────────────
x   x   x   x   x
```

Answer, page 177

136. What word, expression, or name is depicted below?

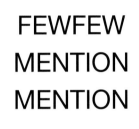

FEWFEW
MENTION
MENTION

Answer, page 200

137. Find a three-digit number containing three different digits where the first digit plus the number formed by the second and third digits, the first digit multiplied by the number formed by the second and third digits, and the sum of the three digits are all perfect squares.

Answer, page 188

138. Which three boys' names are anagrams of one another?

Answer, page 189

139. Five checks by White in four moves (including a double check) followed by a checkmate to solve a puzzle that is more than 500 years old! It was first published by Lucena in 1496.

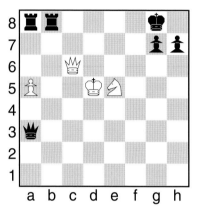

White to play and mate in five.

Answer, page 186

140. Two equal squares, ABCD and DEFG, have the vertex D in common. The angle between the two squares is 60°:

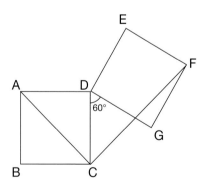

What is the angle ACF?

Answer, page 194

141. Which is bigger?

$$\sqrt{(12 + \sqrt{(12 + \sqrt{(12 + \sqrt{(12 + \dots)})})})}$$

or

$$2 + \sqrt{(2 + \sqrt{(2 + \sqrt{(2 + \sqrt{(2 + \dots)})})})}$$

Answer, page 195

142. What word, expression, or name is depicted below?

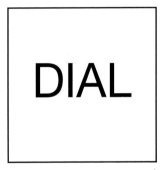

Answer, page 203

143. Find a four-digit number, with four different digits, that is equal to the number formed by its digits in descending order minus the number formed by its digits in ascending order.

Answer, page 178

144. Two candles, one of which was two centimeters longer than the other, were lit for Halloween. The longer and thinner one was lit at 4 P.M. and the shorter but fatter one 15 minutes later. Each candle burned at a steady rate, and by 8 P.M. both were the same length. The thinner one finally burned out at midnight and the fatter one an hour later. How long was each candle originally?

Answer, page 200

145. What word, expression, or name is depicted below?

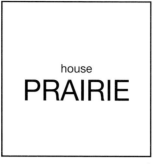

Answer, page 178

146. The following eight numbers can be grouped into four pairs such that the higher of each pair divided by the lower is a number (to an average of five decimal places) of particular mathematical significance.

$$113 \quad 323 \quad 355 \quad 408 \quad 577 \quad 610 \quad 878 \quad 987$$

What are the four pairs?

Answer, page 188

147. The following relationships hold among the ages of the members of a family of four. All ages are integral.

The mother is three times as old as the daughter was when the father was the same age as the mother is now. When the daughter reaches half the age the mother is now, the son will be half as old as the father was when the mother was twice the age the daughter is now. When the father reaches twice the age the mother was when the daughter was the same age as the son is now, the daughter will be four times as old as the son is now. Given that one of their ages is a perfect square, what are the four ages?

Answer, page 195

148. What word, expression, or name is depicted below?

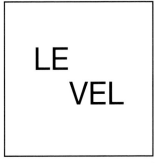

Answer, page 193

149. Any integer from 1 to 112 inclusive can be expressed with four fours, parentheses where necessary, and use of the following seven symbols as required:

$$+ \quad - \quad \times \quad / \quad . \quad ! \quad \sqrt{}$$

All that is asked for here, however, is an expression for 71. The use of other symbols or nonstandard expressions such as $.(\sqrt{4})$ for 0.2 or $\sqrt{\sqrt{\ldots \sqrt{\sqrt{4}}}}$ for 1 is not permitted.

Answer, page 186

150.   *Twice eight are ten of us, and ten but three.*
     Three of us are five. What can we be?
     If this is not enough, I'll tell you more.
     Twelve of us are six, and nine but four.

Answer, page 189

151. In the expression below, each letter represents a different digit:

$$A^5 + B^5 + C^5 + D^5 + E^5 = ABCDE$$

What is ABCDE?

Answer, page 177

152. This self-mate in four was first published by William Shinkman in the *Chess Player's Chronicle* in 1883.

In a fit of kindness, White decides she wants Black to win and offers her resignation. Black turns down White's offer by announcing that he thinks the game should be played to the finish.

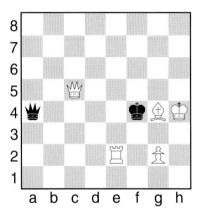

White then forced Black to mate her in four moves anyway. How does White do this?

Answer, page 184

153. What word, expression, or name is depicted below?

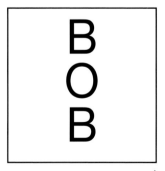

Answer, page 186

154. A professor asked four students how long each of them had been studying. One of the students replied: "We have all been studying a whole number of years, the sum of our years of studying is equal to the number of years you have been teaching, and the product of our years of studying is 180."

"I'm sorry," replied the professor after some thought, "but that doesn't give me enough information."

"Yes, you're right," agreed another of the students. "But if we told you whether any of us were into double figures in our years of study, then you could answer your question."

How long had each of the four been studying?

Answer, page 174

155. In how many different ways can the 16 chess pieces be arranged on one side of a chess board for the start of a game of chess? For example, the two rooks can switch places, and any two of the eight pawns can be swapped and still leave the standard starting position.

Answer, page 198

156. What word, expression, or name is depicted below?

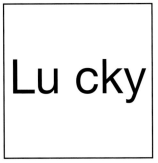

Answer, page 187

157. In an athletics contest between the army, the navy, and the air force, each team entered three athletes in a particular race. The winning athlete scored eight points, the runner-up seven, third place six, and so on down to none for last place.

Once the race was run, the judges needed a photograph to separate the first two army men to finish. A member of the navy's team finished last. When the points were totaled, all three teams were found to have the same score.

Find by team the order in which the nine athletes finished.

Answer, page 183

158. What word, expression, or name is depicted below?

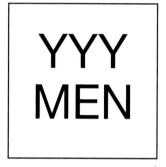

Answer, page 194

159. In a game of chess, Black has agreed to mirror White's first three moves. White promptly mates Black on the fourth move. What were White's moves?

Answer, page 190

160. Which day of the week has an anagram?

Answer, page 182

161. Heather left her hotel room between 7 and 8 P.M. and glanced at her watch. When she next looked at her watch it appeared as if the hour and minute hands had changed places. In fact, it was now between 10 and 11 P.M. Exactly how long ago had she left her room?

Answer, page 189

162. One for the children: Would you rather a tiger chased you or a zebra?

Answer, page 197

163. What word, expression, or name is depicted below?

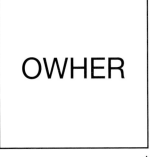

Answer, page 192

164. Find a 3×3 magic square in which the following properties are true:

• The sum of each row, column, and long diagonal is 111.
• Each cell has a number with no factors other than one and itself.
• Each cell is different.

As a hint, you should start by figuring out the center square.

Answer, page 179

165. Both my father and my father's grandfather were born in years that can be expressed as $m^n - n^m$, where m and n are both integers. In which years were they born?

Answer, page 178

166. What word, expression, or name is depicted below?

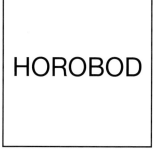

Answer, page 190

167. A, B, C, and D each represent a different word or phrase, and they have a common theme. What are the four words or phrases and what is the theme?

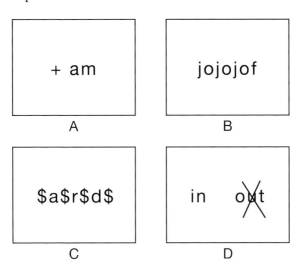

Answer, page 219

168. In the following list of commonly known words, you are given the central letters. Each word begins and ends with the same two letters in the same order. How many words can you complete?

1. ****ca****   2. ****bl****   3. ****eepi****   4. ****adac****

5. ****ur****   6. ****gib****   7. ****risco****   8. ****epsa****

Answer, page 218

169.

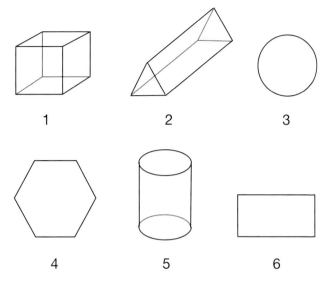

1   2   3

4   5   6

Thinking laterally, which of the following are the seventh and eighth shapes in the series above?

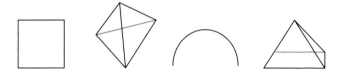

Answer, page 220

170. Find a ten-digit number that:

- can be described as having m digits between the m's, n digits between the n's, and so on, and
- whose first digit is a prime number, the two-digit number formed by its second and third digits is a prime number, the three-digit number formed by its fourth, fifth, and sixth digits is three times a prime number, and the four-digit number formed by its last four digits is also a prime number.

Answer, page 220

171. How can a horseshoe be cut into six pieces with two straight cuts? There are three different ways.

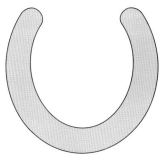

Answer, page 210

172. A, B, C, and D each represent a different word or phrase, and they have a common theme. What are the four words or phrases and what is the theme?

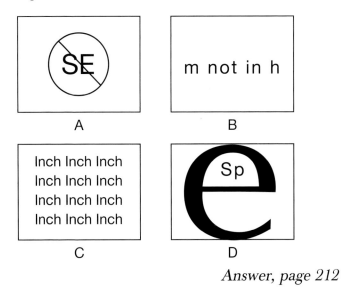

Answer, page 212

173. What two-word phrase could form the first and fourth rows of the diagram so that each column contains a four-letter word?

S	E	O	A	L	O
E	A	T	C	S	E

174. In an international soccer tournament, the scores in a certain round were as follows:

Argentina	0	N. Ireland	0
Belgium	1	Wales	4
England	0	Scotland	1
France	1	Spain	2
Germany	1	Brazil	1
Italy	3	Denmark	1
Peru	2	Cameroon	0
Poland	?	Portugal	?

Each score is related to the name of the corresponding country. Crack the code to figure out what the score was in the final match.

Answer, page 228

175. Complete the grid using all the letters below so that each row and column containing two or more squares is a word when read from left to right or from top to bottom.

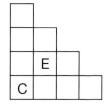

A D E F I N S T

Answer, page 223

176. Each of these crossword clues is a full anagram of the answer.

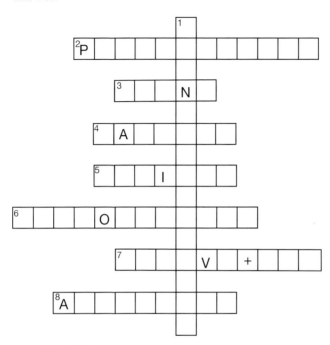

ACROSS

2 I hire parsons (12)

3 On tip (5)

4 Dates up (4,3)

5 Is a lane (2,5)

6 Here come dots (3,5,4)

7 Eleven + two (6+3)

8 Must anger (9)

DOWN

1 No untidy clothes (3,6,6)

Answer, page 223

177. A, B, C, and D each represent a different word or phrase, and they have a common theme. What are the four words or phrases and what is the theme?

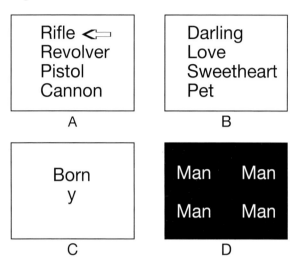

A	B
Rifle ⇐	Darling
Revolver	Love
Pistol	Sweetheart
Cannon	Pet

C	D
Born y	Man Man Man Man

Answer, page 218

178. The answer to the first of these is "29 days in February in a leap year." Complete the rest.

29 D in F in a L Y

12 S of the Z

7 W of the A W

54 C in a D (with the J)

32 D F, at which W F

18 H on a G C

4 Q in a G

14 P in a S

Answer, page 211

179. There are five men in five houses. Each man comes from a different town (all genuine names), has a different pet, and supports a different rugby team. From the following clues, determine which man supports the Waratahs and, if different, which man has a kea.

The five houses are in a row and each is a different color.

The man who has the kangaroo lives next to the man from Woy Woy.

Mr. Brown supports the Brumbies.

The man from Wagga Wagga lives in the blue house.

Mr. Green lives in the mauve house.

The man from Bong Bong has a kookaburra.

Mr. White comes from Aka Aka.

Mr. Gray lives on the left in the first house.

The red house is to the right of and adjacent to the yellow house.

The man from Peka Peka supports the Hurricanes.

The man who has a koala lives next door to the man from Wagga Wagga.

Mr. Black has a kiwi.

The man in the middle house supports the Sharks.

The man in the red house supports the Crusaders.

The maroon house is next to Mr. Gray's house.

Answer, page 214

180. Find a four-digit number that is equal to the square of the sum of the number formed by its first two digits and the number formed by its last two digits, and is exactly 1,000 different from another four-digit number with the same property.

Answer, page 213

181. A, B, C, and D each represent a different word or phrase, and they have a common theme. What are the four words or phrases and what is the theme?

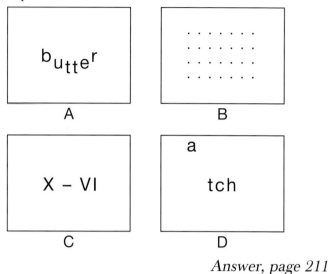

Answer, page 211

182. Two lists of words have been created. Embedded in one list are the 26 letters of the alphabet in their correct order. Embedded in the other list are the 26 letters of the alphabet in reverse order.

The alphabet (forward or backward, as appropriate) has been removed from each list, and the spaces between words have been closed up. In each case the following letters remain:

DOEBOSITELEROEUIUSIGUATGLIEAEST

All the words in the original two lists have at least three letters, and each word in each list includes at least one letter from the above string and at least one letter of the alphabet that was subsequently removed.

Find two lists of words—one containing the 26 letters of the alphabet in their correct order and the second containing the 26 letters in reverse alphabetical order—that meet these conditions.

Answer, page 212

183. The Golden Bay Dining Tour itinerary includes six dinners. Five holidaymakers following this itinerary are all at different stages of the tour. One holidaymaker has dined once so far, and the other four have dined two, three, four, and five times. The dining itinerary begins and ends with dinner at The Old School Cafe, and the four dinners between are at four other restaurants and always in the same order.

From this information and the information below, determine where each holidaymaker comes from, the name of the restaurant at which the holidaymaker last dined, and the name of the restaurant at which the holidaymaker will be dining next.

1. Ann, who is not from Christchurch, will dine next at the Farewell Spit Cafe.
2. Ben does not come from Auckland.
3. Cathy, who last dined at Milliways Restaurant, will not be dining at the Collingwood Tavern next.
4. David is not from Auckland or Dunedin, and dined last at somewhere other than the Collingwood Tavern.
5. Emma comes from Hamilton.
6. The next person to dine at the Wholemeal Cafe did not last dine at the Collingwood Tavern.
7. Ben, the person from Christchurch, the person who last dined at the Farewell Spit Cafe, and the person who will next dine at Milliways Restaurant are four of the five holidaymakers.
8. Neither the person from Wellington nor the person from Dunedin will be dining next at the Collingwood Tavern.

Answer, page 235

184. Although this puzzle seems easy when you hear the answer, few people are able to get all four answers right the first time. In fact, three out of four can be considered a very good score. Name the northernmost, southernmost, easternmost, and westernmost states of the U.S.A.

Answer, page 211

185. A calendar comprises a stand and two printed cubes. Each day both cubes are positioned in the stand to read the day's date, which can of course be any number from 01 to 31. How are the numbers arranged on the cubes?

Answer, page 213

186. A, B, C, and D each represent a different word or phrase, and they have a common theme. What are the four words or phrases and what is the theme?

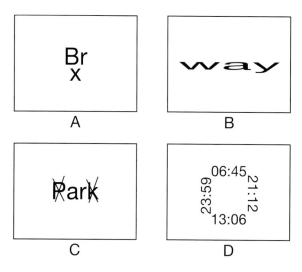

Answer, page 214

187. Tennis is a sport in which you can you take a container that is half full of balls, add another ball, and still have a container that is half full. True or false?

Answer, page 215

188. What is the missing number?

9   22   24   12   ___   4   13

Answer, page 217

189. Each of these crossword clues is a full anagram of the answer.

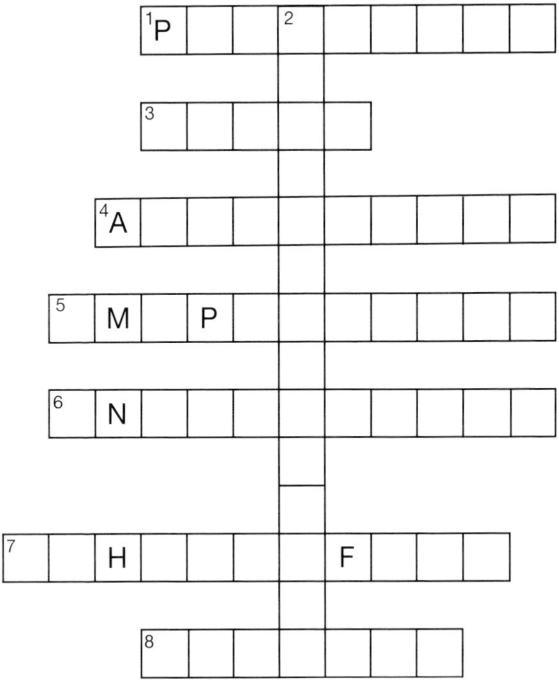

ACROSS

1 Stopped? No (9)

3 The or (5)

4 Moon starer (10)

5 Name for ship (3,8)

6 Tender names (11)

7 Has to pilfer (1,10)

8 They see (3,4)

DOWN

2 No city dust here (3,11)

Answer, page 216

190. A, B, C, and D each represent a different word or phrase, and they have a common theme. What are the four words or phrases and what is the theme?

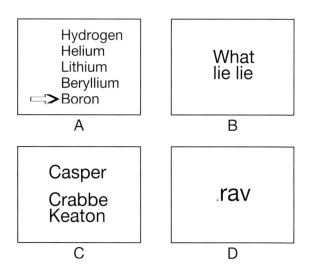

Answer, page 223

191. The first ten natural numbers have been arranged into columns according to a certain rule, as shown below:

1	4	3
2	5	7
6	9	8
10		

A. The numbers 11 and 12 would appear in the same column as each other, but which one?

B. If the arrangement were continued indefinitely, what would be the final entry in the third column?

Answer, page 214

192. Although at first you may not think so, this paragraph is unusual. A quick study will show that it has capitals, commas, and full stops so that punctuation, as far as I know, is satisfactory. But this paragraph is most unusual, and I would hazard my opinion that you do not know why. Should you look at it backwards, or in a mirror, or both, you will find just rubbish, so obviously that is not a way to a solution. Ability at crosswords and similar things may assist you, but I doubt it. If you still do not know what this paragraph is all about, you could go back and start again, but you should not find it particularly difficult. I warn you to watch for your sanity though, as this paragraph is unnatural. Can you work out why? Good luck!

Answer, page 228

193. Security at Prime Palace is a very straightforward affair. There are no keys, just simple bracelets on which are hung five numbers. Access to sensitive areas is then granted by presenting the bracelet in a way that shows a five-digit prime number. Given that a bracelet can be read clockwise or counterclockwise and there are five numbers to start from, the chances of picking a prime number at random can therefore be as low as one in ten.

Sounds simple? Well, as an extra check, you are asked to swap your bracelet for one of the same color at every door, so you need to know for your color the full set of possible prime numbers.

Although the system worked well for many years, it was almost abandoned when the queen remarried. The new king simply could not remember his numbers! He therefore was given a special bracelet that always produced a prime however it was presented, and he was never asked to swap bracelets.

What numbers were on the king's bracelet?

Answer, page 217

194. Prime Palace (see puzzle 193 above) now wants to move to a six-figure system. Will there be a suitable new bracelet for the king?

Answer, page 216

195. Place the numbers from 1 to 19 in the diagram in such a way that the numbers in each of the 15 straight lines of small hexagons have the same total, namely 38. It is not easy, but it can be done!

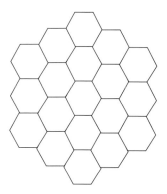

Answer, page 220

196. A, B, C, and D each represent a different word or phrase, and they have a common theme. What are the four words or phrases and what is the theme?

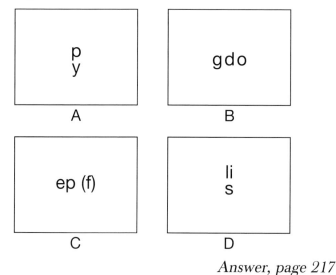

Answer, page 217

197. Readers are no doubt familiar with word search puzzles, where various (usually related) words are hidden in an array and the puzzle is simply to find them. The words may run horizontally, vertically, or diagonally, may run in either direction, or may overlap, but they must run in a straight line. Often there are letters in the array that are not used.

Construct a word search puzzle using the words ONE, TWO, THREE, FOUR, FIVE, SIX, SEVEN, EIGHT, NINE, TEN, ELEVEN, and TWELVE in the grid below.

When completed, the diagram below will have just one unused letter.

Answer, page 215

198. The name of which country includes both a "q" and a "z"?

Answer, page 217

199. Can it be said that the six words below are in alphabetical order?

almost   belt   dirt   know   jot   most

Answer, page 217

200. Zoe's solitaire board consists of 28 holes set out in a triangle as shown in the diagram. The game starts with a peg in every hole except the central one (shaded in the diagram) and is played in the usual way. Each move consists of jumping a peg over an adjacent peg into a hole, with the peg over which the jump is made then being removed from the board. The aim is to be left with only one peg on the board.

Through trial and error, Zoe has convinced herself that the puzzle is impossible. Can you help her prove this?

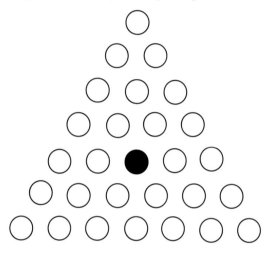

Answer, page 218

201. X and XSUM are two variables related to each other as follows:

XSUM equals the total of the digits comprising X
X equals (XSUM)³

One solution is XSUM = 8 and X = 512, where XSUM as well as X is a cube. Trivial solutions where XSUM as well as X are cubes are X = XSUM = 0 and X = XSUM = 1. Given that there is one more solution where XSUM is a cube than when XSUM is not a cube, how many solutions are there?

Answer, page 219

202. What were the relationships of the people mentioned in the following epitaph?

Two husbands with their two wives
Two grandmothers with their two granddaughters
Two fathers with their two daughters
Two mothers with their two sons
Two maidens with their two mothers
Two sisters with their two brothers
But only six in all lie buried here
All born legitimate, from incest clear.

Answer, page 213

203. A, B, C, and D each represent a different word or phrase, and they have a common theme. What are the four words or phrases and what is the theme?

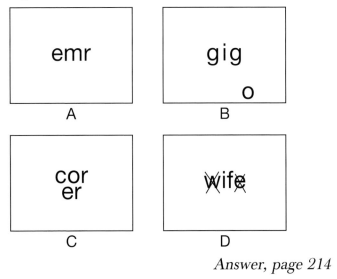

Answer, page 214

204. What three letters should be placed in the three empty circles in order that the longest possible word (which may be more than eight letters long) can be spelled out by reading around the circles? You can choose your starting position and whether to read the letters clockwise or counterclockwise.

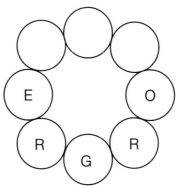

Answer, page 236

205. A carpenter has a solid cube of wood, each edge of which is twelve inches long. He wishes to cut the block in two in such a way that the new face on each of the two pieces can then be trimmed to a square of maximum possible size. Where should he make the cut?

Answer, page 213

206. Each word in the following list is an anagram of a country, but with one letter changed. For example, "least" would lead to "Wales," with "w" replaced by "t." What are the countries?

1. empty	5. amenity
2. tiara	6. elegant
3. tribal	7. glacier
4. warden	8. senator

Answer, page 236

207. Jimmy learned in school that $1^2 + 2^2 = 5$ and $3^2 + 4^2 = 5^2$. Hurrying to do his homework, he writes $1^3 + 2^3 + 3^3 = 6^2$ and then $3^3 + 4^3 + 5^3 = 6^3$. Was he right?

Answer, page 211

208. Divide this figure into four parts, with each part being the same size and shape and comprising whole squares only. Each of the four parts should also contain one X and one O, though not necessarily in the same relative positions.

	X			X	O
		O		X	
				X	
		O	O		

Answer, page 219

209. A, B, C, and D each represent a different word or phrase, and they have a common theme. What are the four words or phrases and what is the theme?

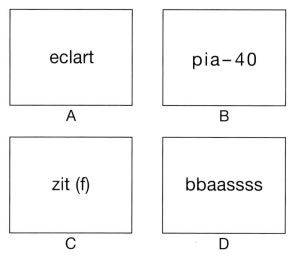

eclart

A

pia−40

B

zit (f)

C

bbaassss

D

Answer, page 223

210. Triangle OAB is formed by three tangents to a circle with center C. Angle AOB = 40°. What is angle ACB?

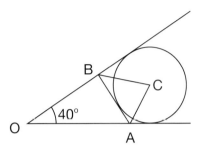

Answer, page 219

211. In the equation below, each letter represents one digit, only, and no letter represents the same digit as any other letter:

$$\text{TIM} \times \text{SOLE} = \text{AMOUNT}$$

Furthermore, and using the same letters to represent the same digits, the difference between LEAST and MOST is ALL. In this puzzle a number may begin with zero; such a zero should be ignored when performing calculations. What digits do the letters stand for?

Answer, page 237

212. Using four 4's, parentheses as necessary, and the following seven symbols as required, find expressions for 73 and 89.

$$+ \quad - \quad / \quad \times \quad . \quad ! \quad \sqrt{}$$

The use of nonstandard expressions such as $.(\sqrt{4})$ for 0.2 or $(\sqrt{\sqrt{\sqrt{\ldots\sqrt{\sqrt{4}}}}})$ for 1 is not permitted.

Answer, page 221

213. An army four miles long steadily advances four miles while a dispatch rider gallops from the rear to the front, delivers a dispatch to the commanding general as he turns, and gallops back to the rear. How far has the rider traveled?

Answer, page 221

214. A crossword puzzle with some puzzling clues:

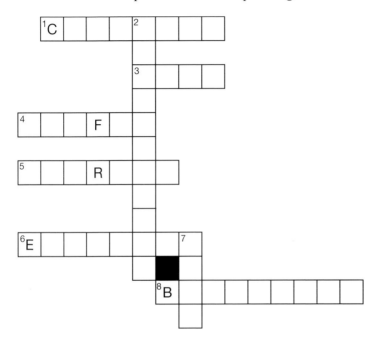

ACROSS

1 A kettle called Ronald (8)

3 Divide or add to make her shorter (4)

4 A word that is an anagram of itself (6)

5 An American film actress from Germany (3,4)

6 Contains the letter "e" three times, but often seen containing just one letter (8)

8 ONMLKJIH (9)

DOWN

2 A rope ends it (11)

7 Cheese made backwards (4)

Answer, page 213

215. "Catchphrase" has six consonants in a row and does not have a y. Find a word that starts with seven consonants in a row, counting y as a consonant, and ends with nine.

Answer, page 212

216. A, B, C, and D each represent a different word or phrase, and they have a common theme. What are the four words or phrases and what is the theme?

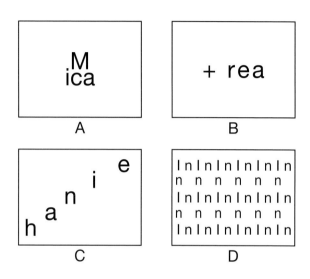

Answer, page 223

217. *If Alan is from New Zealand,*
And Britain's where Rita is from,
Please tell me if you are so able,
The countries of Eric and Don?

Answer, page 224

218. **THIS** × **THAT** × **IT** equals a ten-digit number containing each digit once. If each letter represents a different digit, and **THAT** is a perfect square, what is **THIS**?

Answer, page 228

219. What is the missing letter below?

E O E R E X ? T E N

Answer, page 224

220. The hole for letters in the pillar-box at our local post office is rectangular and wider than it is high. Each side of the hole is an integral number of inches in length, and the area of the hole in square inches is 25 percent greater than the perimeter in inches. What is the width of the hole?

Answer, page 220

221. Find an eight-digit number containing eight different digits that is equal to the square of the sum of the number formed by its first four digits and the number formed by its last four digits.

Answer, page 221

222. Jill has thought of a number between 13 and 1,300, and Jack is doing his best to guess it. Unknown to Jack, Jill is not always truthful.

Jack asks whether the number is below 500.　　　Jill lies.

Jack asks whether the number is a perfect square.　Jill lies.

Jack asks whether the number is a
 perfect cube.　　　　　　　　　　　Jill tells the truth.

Jack then asks whether the second digit is a zero.　Jill lies.

Jack then states the number that he thinks Jill thought of and, not surprisingly, is wrong. From the information above, name Jill's number.

Answer, page 222

223. At work, Alan, Ben, Claire, Dave, Emma, Fiona, Gail, and Henry have their lunch break together. Their lunchroom has four tables against a wall, each for two people.

They decided to have a quiz week where they would each read puzzles over lunch from their favorite puzzle book. In alphabetical order, the eight favorite puzzle books, one per person, were: *Brain Bafflers*, *Crosswords*, *Cryptograms*, *Logic Puzzles*, *Mazes*, *Number Games*, *Probability Paradoxes*, and *Word Search*.

In that week, no two people sat together at lunch more than once. Given that they all lunched together every day unless stated otherwise, determine each person's favorite puzzle book.

Monday

Alan sat beside the reader of *Number Games*.

The *Crosswords* reader was on a diet and skipped the lunch break.

Tuesday

The *Word Search* reader sat beside Gail, and Ben sat beside Emma.

In the evening, Claire left for a week's holiday.

Wednesday

Dave sat beside the *Word Search* reader.

Fiona was ill and so did not go to work that day.

The *Brain Bafflers* reader sat beside Alan, who is not the reader of *Word Search*.

Thursday

The *Mazes* reader was away on business in the morning and missed lunch.

Alan and Emma sat together.

The woman whose favorite puzzle book is *Cryptograms* sat beside Dave.

Friday

Ben took the day off.

Fiona and Dave sat together.

Saturday

The readers of *Number Games* and *Logic Puzzles* sat together.

Answer, page 218

224. A, B, C, and D each represent a different word or phrase, and they have a common theme. What are the four words or phrases and what is the theme?

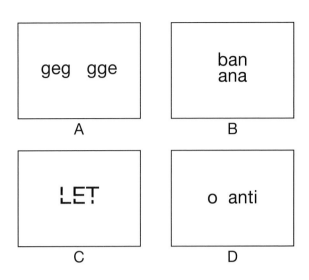

Answer, page 223

225. Two pupils were to be chosen at random from a school register to take part in a competition. The probability that both would be boys was one-third. Before the choice could be made, however, a decision was taken to include pupils from the register of another school in the ballot for the two places. This other school had a register of 1,000 pupils, and the chance that the two selected pupils would both be boys was reduced to one-thirteenth.

How many pupils are on the register of the first school?

Answer, page 226

226. Punctuate the following so that it makes sense:

Time flies you cannot they go too quickly

Answer, page 223

227. Each clue in this crossword leads to two words that are anagrams of each other. For example, the clue "Drums like the Concorde" would give PERCUSSION/SUPERSONIC. Use interlocking letters to determine which word is to be entered in the diagram.

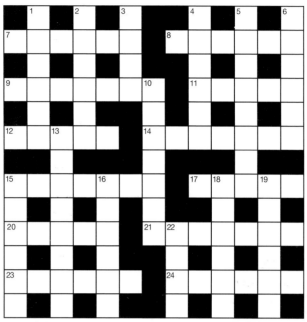

ACROSS

7 Least colorful parts of a flower (6)

8 Confident save (6)

9 Very odd place for hot coals (7)

11 Subsequently change (5)

12 Provide food for a very small quantity (5)

14 Dependent upon where one finds a relieved soldier? (7)

15 Fired for trying to lose pounds (7)

17 Express reaches the top (5)

20 Applauds the top of the head (5)

21 Place: the upper part (7)

23 Removes more than one case of spots (6)

24 Slip away in a dreamy state (6)

DOWN

1 A type of paper tiger, say (6)
2 Sat down and composed (6)
3 Skills of leading performer (4)
4 Enlarge a small part (6)
5 Most impertinent piece of baggage (8)
6 Got to know regular payment (6)
10 Made furious (7)
13 Produce an adolescent, possibly (8)
15 Came out of obsolescence (6)
16 Make known it may be sweaty (6)
18 Pet dog doubled back (6)
19 Tolerates having prejudice (6)
22 Cheese and wine (4)

Answer, page 226

---

228. Construct a chess game in which White moves one piece twice and opens with 1. P–KB3 (see diagram), and Black mates on move five with 5. . . . . N x R mate using his king's knight.

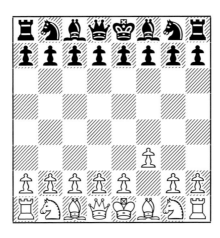

Answer, page 224

229. This is the same as the previous puzzle, but this time the mate in five is with Black's queen's knight.

Answer, page 209

230. Each number from 90 to 99 has been expressed as the product or quotient of two positive integers, neither of which is 1. Each of these integers has, in turn, been expressed as a combination of two integers, and it is these that appear in the diagram below. No number in the diagram begins with 0, and no number appears twice. Capital letters denote "across" numbers, and lowercase letters denote "down" numbers.

A	a	b	B	c	Cd		D	e	f
Eg		F	h	G			Hi		
I		j	J		K	k			l
	m	L		n	Mo		N	p	
Oq			P			Q	r	R	
S			T		U		V		

$$90 = (A - n) \cdot (H / a)$$
$$91 = (e / E) \cdot (r - F)$$
$$92 = (i \cdot V) / (O \cdot T)$$
$$93 = (g / d) \cdot (o - I)$$
$$94 = (G \cdot p) / (B \cdot l)$$

$$95 = (c - j) \cdot (k - M)$$
$$96 = (D \cdot h) \cdot (K \cdot Q)$$
$$97 = (f \cdot P) / (b - C)$$
$$98 = (J / q) \cdot (N / U)$$
$$99 = (R \cdot S) / (L - m)$$

Answer, page 225

231. In a league of four hockey teams, each team played the other three. After all six games had been played, the following league table was prepared:

Team	Goals	
	For	Against
A	4	0
B	2	1
C	1	3
D	2	5

Team D drew one game and lost its other two. What was the score in each of the six games?

Answer, page 216

232. ABC is an equilateral triangle. Point P within the triangle is six inches from A, eight inches from B, and ten inches from C. What is the area of the triangle?

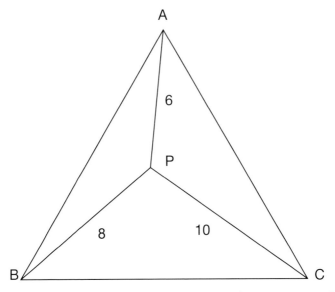

Answer, page 208

233. The answer to the first of these is "24 hours in a day." Complete the rest.

24 H in a D

5 V in the E A

8 L on a S

1,000 W that a P is W

13 S on the A F

14 L in a S

90 D in a R A

9 L of a C

Answer, page 209

234. Benford's Law applies to the terms of the Fibonacci series, the first few of which are shown below:

$$1 \quad 1 \quad 2 \quad 3 \quad 5 \quad 8 \quad 13 \quad 21 \quad 34 \quad \ldots$$

That is, the percentage of numbers in the Fibonacci series beginning with the digit N is log $(1 + 1/N) \times 100\%$. Thus, for example, 30.1% (= log(2) × 100%) of the terms in the Fibonacci series begin with a "1." Benford's Law applies to all sorts of other things too, such as share prices, numbers in old magazine articles, and the drainage areas of rivers.

Prove that the percentage of numbers that are predicted to begin with one of the digits between one and nine using the Benford's Law formula total 100%.

Answer, page 210

235. In how many ways can the numbers from 1 to 9 be arranged in a 3×3 array, such that no number has a smaller number than itself appearing either immediately below or immediately to the right of it?

Answer, page 210

236. Find a 4 × 4 magic square that contains 16 different integers, each of which is divisible only by itself and one. As a start, one row has already been completed.

As a further hint, the middle four squares have the same total as the rows, columns, and long diagonals.

53	11	37	1

Answer, page 232

237. You have several identical crystals that will shatter if dropped from a certain height or above, but which will remain unscathed if dropped from any height lower than this.

You are in a building that has 106 floors. You have already discovered that a crystal dropped from a window on floor 106 will shatter, but you want to know the lowest floor from which you can drop a crystal so that it will shatter.

You could test one floor at a time starting from floor one, but to save time you want a quicker way than this, so long as no more than two more crystals will be shattered during the testing. From which floor should you make the first drop, and what is the maximum number of drops you will require?

Answer, page 227

238. Using three fours, parentheses where necessary, and the eight symbols below as required, find expressions for 119, 268, and 336.

$$+ \quad - \quad \times \quad / \quad . \quad ! \quad \sqrt{} \quad \Sigma$$

The expression Σn denotes the sum of the first n integers, so $\Sigma 4 = 10$. The use of symbols other than those shown, or nonstandard expressions such as $.(\sqrt{4})$ for 0.2, $.(\Sigma 4)$ for 0.1, or $\sqrt{}\sqrt{}\sqrt{}...\sqrt{}\sqrt{4}$ for 1, is not permitted.

Answer, page 228

239. In this crossword, clues are of four different types: synonyms, antonyms, anagrams, and a fourth type that must be determined.

ACROSS

1 Pistol
5 Venomous
10 Pause
11 Coordinate
13 Tear
14 Airs
15 Realize
16 Adze
17 Discern
18 Storm
21 Pleases
24 Dialect
26 Vent
27 Confirm
29 Tail
30 Idol
32 Infidelity
33 Common
34 Patriot
35 Ransom

DOWN

2 Bill
3 Abolish
4 Diet
6 Richest
7 Cater
8 Success
9 Sparing
12 Spoil
16 Young
19 Item
20 Spread
21 Weirdo
22 Bent
23 Sways
24 Urban
25 General
28 Devil
31 Dear

Answer, page 217

240. A New York insurance company has six account managers, each of whom has a different number of children from none to five. Deduce from the following who has what number of children, the account each manages, and where each lives.

1. Angela has two more children than the manager from Manhattan, who has one more child than the fire manager.
2. The marine manager has two more children than the manager from Queens, who has one more child than Enid.
3. The manager from Staten Island has two more children than Dick, who has one more child than the automotive manager.
4. Chloe has three more children than the property manager.
5. The liability manager has more children than the manager from the Bronx, who is not Enid.
6. The manager from Manhattan, who is not the automotive manager, is not Chloe.
7. Enid is not the property manager, and Fred is not the marine manager.
8. The manager from New Jersey may or may not be Brian.
9. The manager from Brooklyn is not the liability manager, but might be the aviation manager.

Answer, page 225

241. A businessman usually travels home each evening on the same train, and his wife leaves home by car just in time to pick him up from the station. One day he caught an earlier train, and having forgotten to tell his wife, he walked to meet the car and was then driven straight home, arriving ten minutes earlier than normal.

The businessman's wife drove at a steady 36 mph each way. Had she been a faster driver, averaging 46 mph, then perhaps surprisingly they would have arrived home just eight minutes earlier rather than ten. This is because being a faster driver and planning to arrive at the station at the same time, the wife would have left home later.

How early was the train?

Answer, page 227

242. In this crossnumber puzzle, each number to be entered in the diagram is clued by the number of factors that it has. In this context, both 1 and the number itself are counted as factors. Thus, if 14 were one of the numbers to be entered in the diagram, its clue would be 4, since 14 has four factors (1, 2, 7, and 14).

There is one condition: in the finished diagram, each of the digits from 0 to 9 must appear twice.

Capital letters denote across answers and lowercase letters denote down answers. No answer begins with a zero.

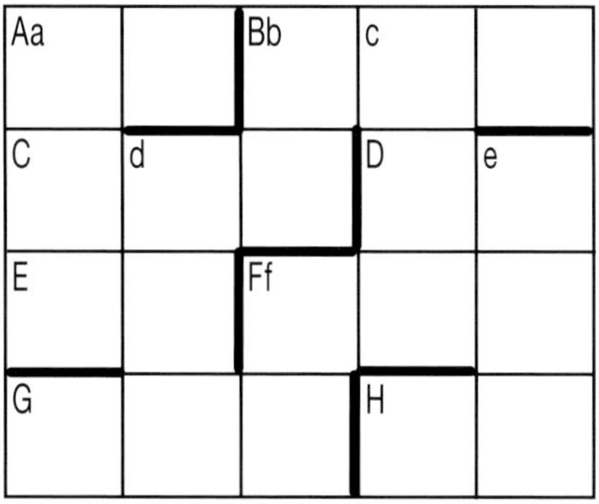

ACROSS		DOWN	
A	8	**a**	15
B	12	**b**	2
C	2	**c**	9
D	6	**d**	18
E	6	**e**	8
F	24	**f**	10
G	14		
H	6		

Answer, page 228

243. A, B, C, and D each represent a different word or phrase, and they have a common theme. What are the four words or phrases and what is the theme?

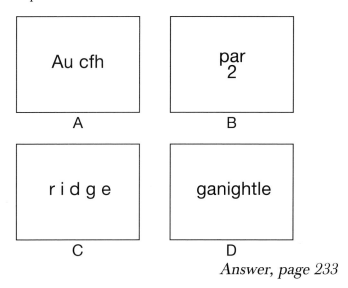

A

par
2

B

r i d g e

C

ganightle

D

244. P and Q are five-digit numbers that between them contain all ten digits, as does their product, P × Q. If P = 54,321, what is Q?

Answer, page 232

245. Tires on Cathy's car last 18,000 miles on the front or 22,000 miles on the back. She has a new set of five tires (including the spare) that she intends to rotate so they can all be replaced at the same time.

   A. Assuming no punctures or blowouts, how far can she drive with five tires?

   B. Which tires will need to be changed and at what distances if the number of wheel changes she makes is to be kept to a minimum?

Answer, page 221

246. Heather and Lynsey are playing a game of Boxes and have reached the position shown. The object of the game is to complete the most boxes as signified by the initials inside. The rules are that players take turns by adding to the grid a horizontal or vertical line of unit length, and that they have a compulsory extra turn whenever they complete a box. It is Lynsey's turn to play. How can she win?

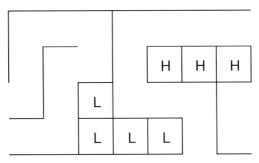

Answer, page 230

247. Samos Farm has four straight sides, and its diagonally opposite corners are joined by two straight roads that run north-south and east-west. The lengths of the sides of the farm and the distances between the crossroads and the four corners are all different, and each is an exact number of chains. (An old-fashioned measure of distance that equals 22 yards.)

Given that one side is 35 chains long and that ten square chains make an acre, what is the farm's area measured in acres?

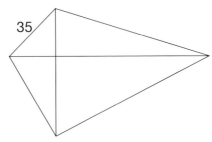

Answer, page 229

248. Here is a "proof" that all triangles are isosceles. Can you spot the flaw?

Begin with any triangle ABC. Let the bisector of angle A meet the perpendicular bisector of BC at O. The diagrams show O inside and outside the triangle, respectively. Let E and F be the feet of the perpendiculars from O to AB and AC.

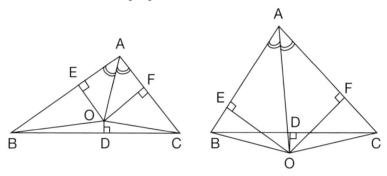

AFO is congruent to AEO, so AE = AF and OE = OF.

BDO is congruent to CDO, so OB = OC.

Thus OEB is congruent to OFC, and EB = FC.

Now, AE = AF and EB = FC, so AE + EB = AF + FC.

Therefore, AB = AC and ABC is isosceles.

Answer, page 235

249. Which two 10-digit numbers, each containing one of each digit, have square roots whose digits are the reverse of one another?

Answer, page 231

250. Find a five-digit palindromic number (a number that equals itself when read backward) that has a remainder of 9 when divided by 10, a remainder of 8 when divided by 9, a remainder of 7 when divided by 8, and so on, and whose digits are all odd.

Answer, page 231

251. The diagram below shows an arrangement of six wooden matches that makes eight triangles.

Without breaking the matches but using lateral thinking, rearrange the six matches to make eight squares.

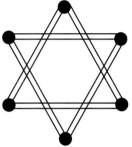

Answer, page 231

252. A, B, C, and D each represent a different word or phrase, and they have a common theme. What are the four words or phrases and what is the theme?

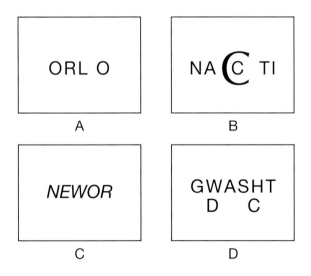

Answer, page 227

253. Place three letters in the three empty circles in order that the longest possible word (which may be more than eight letters long) can be spelled out by reading around the circles. You can choose your starting position and whether to read the letters clockwise or counterclockwise.

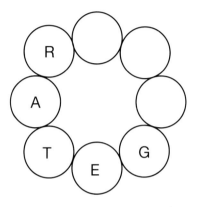

Answer, page 221

254. If Black were to play in the position shown, the game would finish immediately, in stalemate. But White is to play, and he can win in just three moves; how?

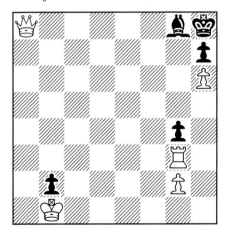

Answer, page 232

255. In this crossnumber puzzle, none of the numbers to be entered in the diagram begins with a zero.

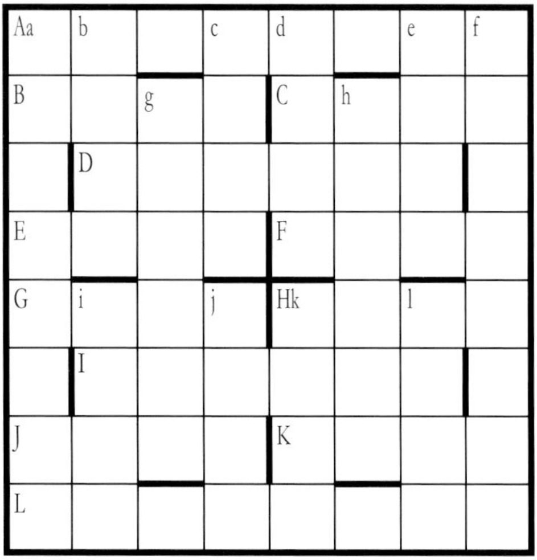

Aa	b		c	d		e	f
B		g		C	h		
	D						
E				F			
G	i		j	Hk		l	
	I						
J				K			
L							

ACROSS	DOWN
A Multiple of j	**a** c·d
B Square	**b** Square
C 1 – d	**c** Square
D Fifth power	**d** Multiple of F
E Fourth power	**e** Twice a prime
F Factor of d	**f** Multiple of j
G Square	**g** Square
H Square	**h** Sixth power
I Sixth power	**i** Prime
J Multiple of c	**j** Cube
K i – 2b	**k** Square
L Multiple of E	**l** C + d

Answer, page 231

256. Complete the grid using all the letters below so that each row and column containing two or more squares is a word when read from left to right or from top to bottom:

A C C E E E H L N O W

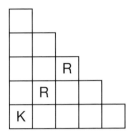

Answer, page 236

257. There are six symmetrical ways in which dots can be placed in 16 different squares in an 8 × 8 array such that every row, column, and diagonal (not just the main diagonals from corner to corner) is either empty or has exactly two dots in it. The solution shown below is one such arrangement, and is also symmetrical when divided in half diagonally from top left to bottom right.

Can you find the one solution (ignoring rotations and reflections) that is not symmetrical?

Answer, page 232

258. This crossword—part jigsaw puzzle—is made from the 28 jigsaw pieces shown below. Where some of the letters on the jigsaw pieces should be turned on their side or upside down (because in the jigsaw, the jigsaw piece itself is turned on its side or upside down), the letters have been shown right side up. To avoid giving unnecessary clues, the pieces have been redrawn to a standard shape.

Identify in the completed crossword the exact position of each individual jigsaw piece.

DI	DE	IA	IR
DA	DR	IP	IS
DP	DS	IE	AP
DD	II	AA	PP
AR	AE	PE	ER
AS	PS	RS	EE
PR	ES	RR	SS

ACROSS

1 Anagram of DIAPERS (7)

4 Another anagram of DIAPERS (7)

7 German villains in Central Russia (2)

9 Raise right, with musical talent (4)

11 Start to play after gym class—it gives you energy (3)

12 Noticed where Pierre is eating dessert (5)

14 The unconscious security guards may ask to see it (2)

15 Another anagram of DIAPERS (7)

16 Caesarean section's region (4)

17 Private eye had backtracked to get pickpocket (3)

DOWN

1 Church areas keep sins from starting (5)
2 Parade is moved to the perfect place (8)
3 Spooky Pennsylvania city makes itself heard (5)
5 In hindsight, that German's upset (3)
6 Dullard to tear after Democrat (4)
8 One who undermines revised papers (6)
10 Gaelic tongue in stanza following introduction (4)
13 By day, spot a close relative (3)
14 Three leaders in Indonesia instigated insurgency (3)

Answer, pages 206-207

259. There are just three clues for this crossnumber:

Every answer is the product of two different primes of equal length.
No answer begins with a zero, and in no answer is a digit repeated.
The digits of the middle six-digit number are in ascending order.

Answer, page 233

260. There was a group of three men. When asked a question, one of the men would always answer truthfully, one would always lie, and the third would lie at random. They know who has which habit, but you do not.

How, in only three questions to which the man being asked can only answer "yes" or "no," can you discover which man has which habit? Each of the three questions can be put to one man only, but it need not be to the same man each time. For example, questions one and two could go to the first man, and question three to the second.

Answer, page 231

261. A rectangular cake is being baked to meet the following requirements:
- The cake can be cut into five rectangular pieces such that each piece has sides that are a whole number of inches long, and
- Sides of the pieces and sides of the original cake all have different measurements.

What is the area of the smallest cake that will meet these requirements?

Answer, page 234

262. A, B, C, and D each represent a different word or phrase, and they have a common theme. What are the four words or phrases and what is the theme?

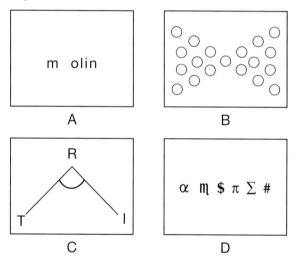

Answer, page 236

263. What property having to do with factorials makes the number 145 interesting?

Answer, page 236

264. Each empty square in this grid is to be filled with a single letter. When read consecutively, the 18 letters spell out a well-known object.

The numbers between the letters provide the only clues. Letting A = 1, B = 2, up to Z = 26, each number is the difference between the adjacent letter values. For example, 4 could separate E and A, B and F, and so on. What is the object?

	12		3		14		1		19	
0	■	13	■	0	■	4	■	14	■	11
	1		16		10		9		6	
11	■	19	■	0	■	3	■	14	■	13
	7		3		13		2		5	

Answer, page 222

265.

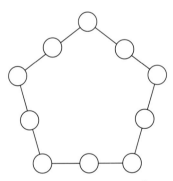

A. Arrange the digits from 0 to 9 in the circles around the pentagon in such a way that the three numbers on each side of the pentagon add up to eleven.

B. Now rearrange the digits in such a way that, starting from a suitable side and moving clockwise, the sums on successive sides are consecutive integers, none of which equals eleven.

Answer, page 228

266. There are nine indistinguishable mince pies. Some mincemeat has been removed from one, chosen at random, and put back in another pie, also chosen at random. Thus, either one pie is light and another heavy by the same amount, or else they all have the same weight.

With four trials using a simple balance, either establish that all mince pies have the same weight or identify the light and heavy ones.

Answer, page 222

267. What two-word phrase could form the first and fourth rows of the diagram, so that each column contains a five-letter word?

U	V	A	L	O
M	E	S	A	D
Y	T	S	E	L

Answer, page 211

268. If all you knew about Britney Spears was that her name was an anagram of "best in prayers," why might you think her parents were not Catholics? (Hint: look for another anagram, this time one word of thirteen letters.)

Answer, page 213

269. David's mother has three children. She also has three coins from the United States and decides to give one to each child.

Penelope is given a penny.

Nicholas is given a nickel.

What is the name of the child who gets the dime?

Answer, page 212

270. The number 153 is interesting for two reasons. The first has something to do with factorials, and the second has to do with cubes. What are these two reasons, and what other three-digit number shares the second property?

271. A, B, C, and D each represent a different word or phrase, and they have a common theme. What are the four words or phrases and what is the theme?

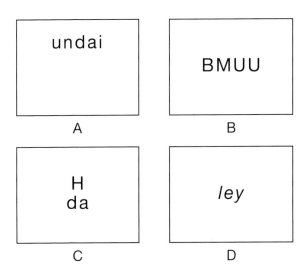

272. Arrange six matches in such a way that each one touches four of the other five.

273. If W = 2, U = 4, V = 5, G = 8, and Y = 20, what does D equal?

274. Seven friends stranded on a desert island start arguing about what day of the week it is.

Andrew thinks that yesterday was Wednesday.

Dave disagrees, saying that tomorrow is Wednesday.

John maintains that the day after tomorrow is Tuesday.

Pete feels sure that yesterday was not Friday.

Fred believes that today is Tuesday.

Mick says that today is not Sunday, Monday, or Tuesday.

Charlie is adamant that it is Tuesday tomorrow.

If just one of them is right, what day of the week is it?

Answer, page 232

275. Which five of these six pieces can be arranged to form a 5 × 5 checkerboard pattern?

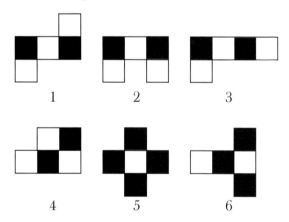

1   2   3

4   5   6

Answer, page 211

276. How should the digits from one to eight be arranged as two four-digit numbers so that the product of the two numbers is **(a)** a minimum and **(b)** a maximum?

Answer, page 216

277. Place a letter in each of the ten spaces such that:

• Five six-letter words, including one country, are formed by reading in a straight line from each of five letters in the outer ring to the ones at the opposite side, and

• The ten letters in the middle circle, read clockwise, spell out the name of another country.

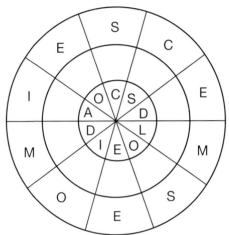

Answer, page 236

278. Four women weighed 105, 110, 115, and 120 pounds. Two weeks ago, Carol announced that she was going on a diet, and the other three immediately decided to join her.

Since starting the diet, no woman's weight has changed by more than five pounds, and all weights are still whole numbers of pounds. Debbie has lost more weight than Miss Easton. Anne weighed ten pounds more than Debbie when they started the diet. Miss Green now weighs ten pounds less than Miss Hope. Miss Frost now weighs seven pounds less than Barbara did before dieting. Miss Hope actually put on weight, but still weighs less than Anne. Barbara has lost more weight than Anne. Miss Easton now weighs four pounds more than Anne.

What are the names and current weights of the four women?

Answer, page 234

279. The segment below is one-sixth of a circle. Dots A and B on the arc divide that arc into thirds. The other two dots, C and D, are two-thirds of the way from the nearest part of the arc to what would have been the center of the circle.

Are the lines AC and BD parallel? If not, on which side of the segment would they meet if they were extended?

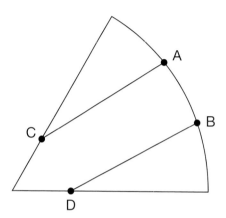

Answer, page 233

280. What number should replace the question mark in the following array?

1	2	3	4	5
1	3	9	21	41
1	4	31	220	1,081
1	5	129	6,949	?

Answer, page 208

281. In a certain fashion show, the exhibits included 36 outfits by Jasper Conran, 35 by Calvin Klein, and 56 by Yves Saint Laurent. How many outfits did Vivienne Westwood exhibit?

Answer, page 233

282. Place the numbers from one to eight in the grid in such a way that each number differs from its neighbors horizontally, vertically, and diagonally by at least two.

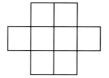

Answer, page 234

283. In this magic square, A, B, and C are single-digit numbers, 2A means twice A, and so on. Every row, column, and both diagonals add up to the same total. What is that total?

2A	C	2C
A+2B	A+B	A
B	3A	2B

Answer, page 235

284. A secretary was asked to organize a mailing to a 10% sample of a company's clients. Rather than just pick 10% of the clients on his mailing list randomly, however, the secretary decided to pick the first client, skip one, pick the next, skip two, pick the next, skip three, pick the next, and so on, until he came to the end of the list. To his surprise, the final client that he picked happened to be the last one on the mailing list. Moreover, as required, he had picked exactly 10% of the total.

How many names were on the mailing list?

Answer, page 234

285. On a regular 8 × 8 chessboard, shown below, only five queens are needed in order to ensure that all unoccupied squares are attacked.

How many queens are needed on an 11 × 11 board?

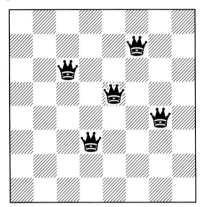

Answer, page 223

286. The diagram below shows five flat interlocked rings lying on the ground. Four are made of a rigid metal; the fifth is made of rubber. Which is the rubber one?

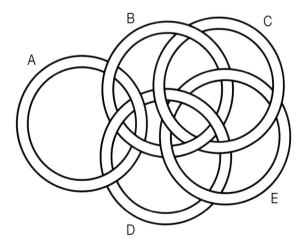

Answer, page 219

287. One leaf has been torn out of a book. The sum of the remaining page numbers is 10,000. What is the last-numbered page in the book, and which leaf is missing?

Answer, page 224

288. The piece below on the left comprises three squares of unit length. What is the smallest rectangle that can be covered with pieces of this shape in a way such that no two pieces form a 2×3 rectangle (as shown below on the right)?

Answer, page 216

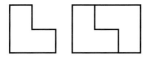

289. The diagram below shows two railway lines with a crossover track. The task for the two engine drivers is to exchange the two wagons on the top track with the two on the bottom track, with the wagons finishing in the same order from left to right as they started. What makes the task difficult is that the usable stretch of straight track at the bottom right will take only two wagons, while the usable stretch at the top right will take only two wagons and an engine. How can the drivers accomplish the task?

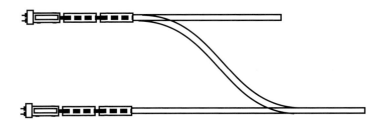

Answer, page 215

290. I ordered four items, the prices of which were $27, $34, $84, and $91. When I went to pay for them, I discovered my son had also ordered one of these items and, quite independently, so had his wife. To save time, I decided to pay for all six items.

Explaining this to the cashier seemed to put him in a state of confusion, because he then entered every price with its digits reversed—so that $27 was entered as $72, for example. However, by a remarkable coincidence, the total turned out to be correct anyway.

How much between them do my son and his wife owe me?

Answer, page 234

291. What three letters should be placed in the three empty circles so that the longest possible word (which may be more than eight letters long) can be spelled out by reading around the circles? You can choose your starting position and whether to read the letters clockwise or counterclockwise.

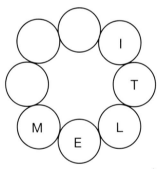

Answer, page 224

292. Emma buys seven items. The prices of the items are all different, and the total cost is $10.71. Emma checks this on her calculator, but inadvertently multiplies the amounts together instead of adding. The result, with correct treatment of decimal points, is also $10.71. What are the prices of the seven items?

Answer, page 232

293. A construction worker was asked to dig a ditch into which a 9" diameter pipe would be laid. He dug a triangular ditch with an angle of 60° to a depth of 12", but as the cross-section shows, this was not deep enough to hide the whole pipe below the surface.

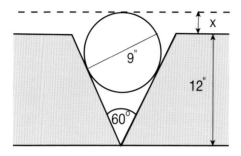

How far above the surface–the distance marked x in the diagram–does the pipe protrude?

Answer, page 212

294. In what way are the letters in the top row different from the letters in the bottom row?

C   I   O   Q   U

B   P   R   T   Y

Answer, page 236

295. An old riddle describes how an explorer, lost in strange territory, set out from her camp, walked a mile south, then a mile east, and then a mile north and found herself back at her camp looking at a bear. The question is then: "What color is the bear?" The answer to this conundrum is "white" because the explorer was at the North Pole, but could the explorer have been anywhere else? If so, where?

Answer, page 236

296. A, B, C, and D each represent a different word or phrase, and they have a common theme. What are the four words or phrases and what is the theme?

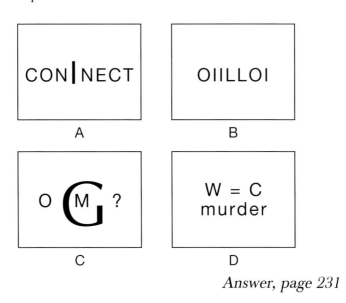

297. Using the integers 1 to 49, construct a 7 × 7 grid where every row, every column, and the two major diagonals add up to 175 (a 7 × 7 magic square), and the grid contains a 5 × 5 and a 3 × 3 magic square.

A start is given in the diagram below.

10						
	19					
		24				
			25			
				26		
					31	
						40

Answer, page 225

298. Three children of different ages share the same birthday. On one of their birthdays, one of their ages was the sum of the other two ages. On another birthday a few years later, the youngest observed that one of their ages was half the sum of the other two ages. When the number of years since the first occasion was half the sum of the ages on the first occasion, one celebrated her 18th birthday. What birthdays were the other two celebrating at this time?

Answer, page 213

299. Which is capable of filling more of the available space—a square peg in a round hole or a round peg in a square hole?

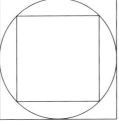

Answer, page 214

300. In this multiplication problem, each digit appears once and once only (so each "X" represents a different digit), and the three-digit number is prime. What are the two numbers that are being multiplied together?

$$\begin{array}{r} X\,X\,X \\ X\,X \\ \hline X\,X\,X\,X\,X \end{array}$$

Answer, page 224

301. Flying over a plantation, the pilot looks down and announces that he can see six rows of four trees. "So that is 24 trees?" his passenger asks. "Actually no," says the pilot, "just half that number."

In what pattern are the trees planted?

Answer, page 209

302. It's easy to make an arithmetical expression equal to 24 from exactly three 8's $(8 + 8 + 8 = 24)$, but an expression for 24 can also be made from exactly three 1's, three 2's, and so on up to three 9's, using standard mathematical symbols: $+$, $-$, $\times$, $\div$, $\sqrt{}$, ! (factorial), decimal point, and $^-$ (repeating decimal). Using no more than three factorial signs in total, find such an expression for each digit from 1 to 9.

Answer, page 246

303. Donald has three daughters of whom he is exceedingly proud. All three are excellent logicians, and in his will he divides his properties among them.

He calls them together and tells them how many properties he owns and that each will inherit a different number of separate properties. He adds that the eldest will inherit the most properties (but not more than ten) and the youngest the fewest (with not fewer than one).

He then whispers in each daughter's ear how many properties she will inherit. After that, he proceeds from the eldest daughter to the youngest, asking each daughter if she can calculate how many properties each of her two sisters will inherit; each daughter replies "No" in turn. He does this a second time, and again all three reply "No." But then, when he asks the question a third time, the eldest daughter says, "Yes; each of the last two answers gave me some information, and I now know how many properties each of us will inherit."

How many properties will each daughter get?

Answer, page 254

304. Can you make a perfect square out of three matchsticks pointing in different directions, without bending or breaking them? (Some lateral thinking will be required!)

Answer, page 260

305. Insert the numbers from 2 to 10 in the nine small circles in such a way that the sum of the numbers appearing around each of the four large circles is the same.

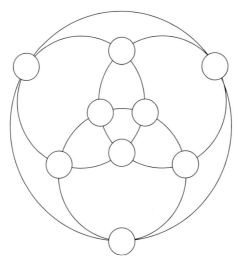

Answer, page 269

306. Hayley has a new sticker album with 250 gaps, each of which requires a particular sticker to fill it. The stickers to fill these gaps are sold individually in opaque sealed packets, so the contents of a packet are not known until the packet is purchased and opened.

Each packet costs 20 cents. But instead of buying every sticker individually, Hayley can write to the publisher of the album and request 25 specified stickers for $12.50, 50 for $25.00, 75 for $37.50, and so on.

Assuming there is an equal chance of a packet containing any of the 250 stickers, how many different individual stickers should Hayley collect before ordering one or more packs of 25 if she wants to minimize the expected cost of collecting a full set of stickers?

Answer, page 267

307. Two identical sets of dominoes, shown below, were used to make the robot on the opposite page. The dominoes in one set were all placed vertically, while the dominoes in the other set were all placed horizontally. The dominoes may, of course, be rotated from the positions shown. Identify the position of each domino in the robot.

Horizontally placed dominoes:

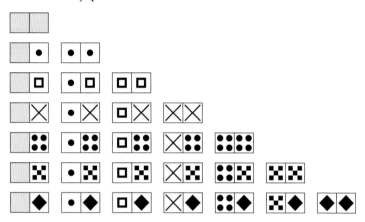

Vertically placed dominoes:

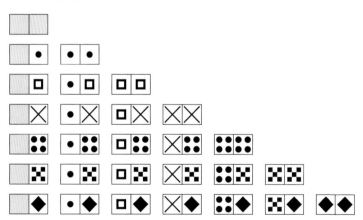

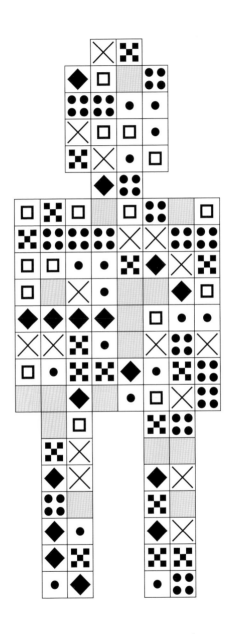

Answer, page 256

308. In this long division problem, all but two of the digits have been replaced with a blank. Can you supply the missing numbers?

```
            _ _ 8 _ _
        _____
  _ _ ) _ _ _ _ _ _ _
        _ _ _
        _ _
        _ _
          _ _ _
          _ _ _
              2
```

Answer, page 249

309. Dozing in the classroom, Sarah awoke to hear her teacher ask, "Sarah, what comes next in this series?" Sarah looked at the blackboard and saw the following:

1, 2, 4, 5, 7, 8 ...

With no time to think, Sarah guessed:

11, 12, 13, 14, 15, 16 ...

After a pause, the teacher congratulated Sarah and moved on to a new topic. Sarah was very relieved, but when the class received its homework, the first question was:

1, 2, 4, 5, 7, 8, 11, 12, 13, 14, 15, 16, ?, ?, ?, ?

What are the next four items in the series?

Answer, page 251

310. Walking down the street, you overhear one person saying to another:

> **"There is too much space between rose
> and and and and and crown."**

How should the sentence be punctuated, and what jobs from the list below might the two people have had?

Architect	Gardener	Moneylender	Taxi driver
Botanist	Historian	News vendor	Undertaker
Courier	Innkeeper	Orthodontist	Veterinarian
Dentist	Jeweler	Plumber	Waiter
Engineer	Karate teacher	Radiologist	Yacht maker
Firefighter	Lawyer	Sign painter	Zoologist

Answer, page 241

311. The local kindergarten is thinking of making posters that show all the different ways of adding together two or more integers from 1 to 9 to make 10. For instance: $1 + 9 = 10$, $9 + 1 = 10$, $2 + 8 = 10$, $8 + 2 = 10$, and $2 + 1 + 2 + 1 + 1 + 2 + 1 = 10$. (Sums that contain the same numbers but in a different order are considered to be different.)

The kindergarten has wall space for ten large posters, and there will be space on each poster for up to 50 possible solutions. Is that enough space for the kindergarten to display every possible solution?

Answer, page 239

312. There are three jugs with capacities of 11, 13, and 17 cups. Each jug contains 9 cups of water. By pouring from jug to jug (and not spilling any water), how can you measure exactly 8 cups of water?

Answer, page 247

313. What word, expression, or name is depicted below?

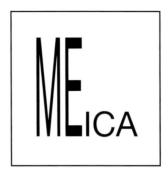

Answer, page 265

314. While playing unattended one day, Thomas decided to build larger cubes out of a box of individual sugar cubes. So, emptying out the box onto the floor and using the sugar cubes as if they were building blocks, Thomas made three larger, solid cubes, with no sugar cubes left over.

At this point the family dog bounded into the room and sent the sugar cubes flying in all directions. The dog then picked up one of the sugar cubes in his mouth and left, crunching noisily.

Knowing he would be blamed for the mess if he didn't clean it up, Thomas picked up the remaining sugar cubes. Once he had done this, however, the temptation to keep playing with them proved too strong, and he began building again. This time he built two cubes rather than three, and again no sugar cubes were left over.

What is the smallest number of sugar cubes that could have been in the box when Thomas started playing with them?

Answer, page 262

315. You're probably familiar with puzzles like "12 = M. in a Y." where the goal is to identify the original phrase (12 = months in a year). The puzzle below is similar, but you are asked to provide the numbers as well. On the first line, for instance, 1,001 (Arabian Nights) – 1,000 (words that a picture is worth) = 1 (wheels on a unicycle).

A.N.	– W. that a P. is W.	= W. on a U.
A.M.	– F. on a P. of G.	= S. to E.S.
D. in F. in a L.Y.	– Y. of M. in a S.A.	= S. in a D. of C.
G. in a H.T.	+ R. on the O.F.	= L. on a S.
N. on a D.	– Q. in a G.	= O. in a P.
H. on a G.C.	+ D. in a F.	= D.F. at which W.F.
D. in a R.A.	– L. of the A.	= S. on a C.

Hint: the numbers on the right form a series.

Answer, page 245

316. A circular road is 31 miles long. There are six gas stations on the road, and it so happens that for every distance from 1 mile, 2 miles, 3 miles, and so on up to 30 miles, there are two gas stations which are that distance apart from each other on the road.

The simplified map below (not to scale) shows the two stations that are one mile apart. Can you determine the positions of the other four gas stations?

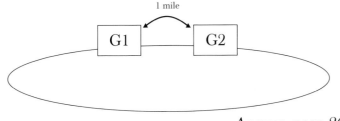

Answer, page 269

317. Each clue in the crossword below takes the form of a number. This number is equal to the product of the values of the letters in the corresponding word, where the value of a letter is equal to its position in the alphabet; thus A = 1, B = 2, C = 3, D = 4, and so on up to Z = 26. The clue for, say, RARE would therefore be $18 \times 1 \times 18 \times 5 = 1{,}620$.

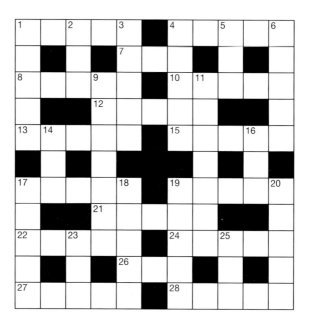

ACROSS				DOWN			
1	1,536	17	14,040	1	17,100	14	810
4	257,040	19	420	2	80	16	1,725
7	3,675	21	23,400	3	9,800	17	42,768
8	720	22	831,600	4	101,250	18	14,820
10	8,820	24	145,800	5	5,292	19	32,400
12	7,560	26	300	6	519,840	20	2,160
13	151,200	27	1,436,400	9	2,268,000	23	1,400
15	228,000	28	6,825	11	567,000	25	1,350

Answer, page 253

318. After leaving the shopping mall, a shopper decided to walk home. (Her home is somewhere on the map below, but is not shown.) She wanted to take as short a route as possible, and she knew she could set off in either direction to achieve this. So she tossed a coin to determine which way she would go.

MALL

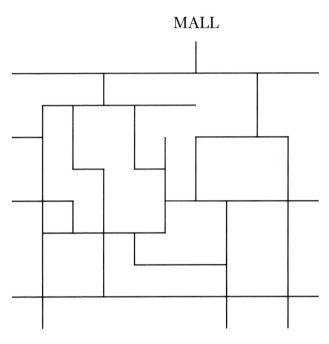

After completing more than half her journey, she reached the intersection where her favorite cafe is situated, and popped in for a coffee. When she left the cafe, it was once again the case that she could set off in either of two directions and still travel the shortest distance to complete her journey home.

Where is the cafe, and where does the shopper live?

Answer, page 259

319. The square of 567 is 321,489, and these two numbers contain each of the digits from 1 to 9 once and once only between them. What other three-digit number and its square have this property?

Answer, page 255

320. A hexagonal plot of land contains six houses as shown below. The six homeowners have agreed that they would like to erect fences to subdivide the whole plot into equal plots for each of them, with each house naturally being on its own plot of land. One of the homeowners pointed out that this could be done by dividing the plot into six congruent (but irregular) pentagons. Where would the fences have to be erected to achieve this?

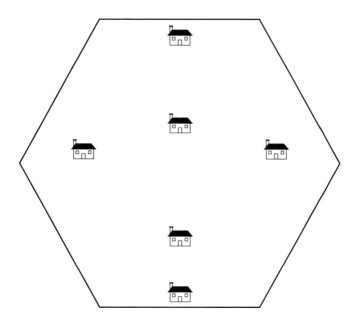

Answer, page 257

321. What is the smallest number that leaves a remainder of 1 when divided by 2, a remainder of 2 when divided by 3, a remainder of 3 when divided by 4, and so on up to a remainder of 17 when divided by 18?

Answer, page 271

322. Without using a calculator or computer, can you find two integers whose squares add up to exactly 100,000?

Once you've done that, do the same for 1,419,857, given that the only prime factor for this number is 17.

Answer, page 247

323. All the digits in the following multiplication problem have been replaced with letters. (A letter always represents the same digit throughout the problem.) Can you reconstruct the original multiplication?

TWO × TWO = THREE

Answer, page 250

324. A number of identical planes, each of which has a tank that will hold just enough fuel to travel exactly halfway around the world, are all based on a small island. If the planes can only refuel from the island or from another plane of their fleet, what is the smallest number of planes that would be required for one plane to complete a great circle around the world, with each plane involved in the maneuver returning safely to the island? Assume that planes can refuel and transfer fuel instantaneously, and that all planes travel at the same constant speed.

Answer, page 263

325. When Rachel looked at the board displaying the hymn numbers of the three carols to be sung at the Christmas Eve service, she was struck by the following:

- Each of the digits from 1 to 9 appeared on the board.
- Each number was a three-digit prime.

Given that the sum of the carols' numbers was less than 1,000, what were the numbers of the carols?

Answer, page 241

326. The set of whole numbers has been split into two groups according to a particular rule; the first ten numbers in each group are shown below.

1	4
2	5
3	9
6	11
7	12
8	13
10	14
15	18
16	19
17	20

The number 100 is also in the second group. In which group does 1,000,000 belong?

Answer, page 243

327. Which four-digit number is equal to its first digit to the power of its second digit, multiplied by its third digit to the power of its fourth digit?

Answer, page 266

328. Two men share the plot of land that their houses are built on. They have agreed to divide the land equally (with each owning the piece of land that his house is built on), but are not sure how best to divide the rest. Since they know you're a puzzle expert, they turn to you.

The diagram below shows the area in question, with the two houses marked in black. Where should the dividing fence be erected so that the two pieces of land *excluding* the houses are equal in area and have the same shape? (Rotations and reflections of a shape are considered to be equivalent.)

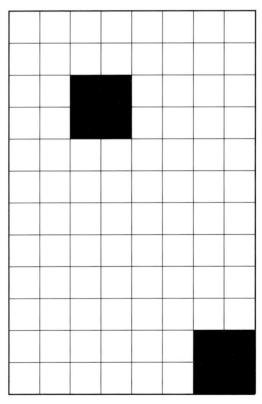

Answer, page 245

329. A pilot wants to begin his plane's descent at point D, but he is told by air traffic control to maintain his altitude and fly directly north. After six minutes of flying, the plane is directly above the control tower (point C). The pilot is then told to fly northwest for three minutes before turning at point T and heading back the thirty miles to point D.

This holding pattern is repeated a few times until the pilot is instead instructed to turn 90 degrees to the left upon arriving at point D. Thirty miles later (at point B), the plane is directed back to the point directly above the control tower.

Assuming that the plane has a constant speed throughout and that the time lost in turning is immaterial, how long does it take the plane to fly from point B to point C?

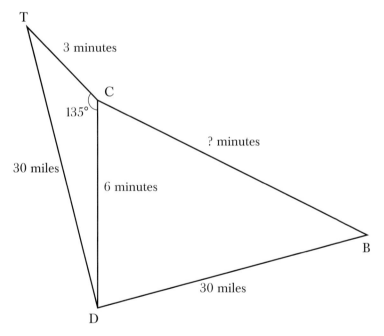

Answer, page 248

330. Find the triangle with the shortest perimeter where:

    a) The sides are of different integral lengths.
    b) The area is a perfect square.

To determine the area of the triangle, use Hero's formula (shown below); let the lengths of the sides be *a*, *b*, and *c*, and let *s* be half the perimeter, or ½(*a* + *b* + *c*):

$$\text{Area of triangle} = \sqrt{[s(s - a)(s - b)(s - c)]}$$

Answer, page 257

331. There is a well-known person whose name, when entered into the first and fourth rows of the diagram below, will spell four-letter words in all six columns. Who is it?

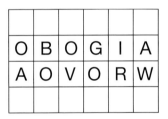

Answer, page 240

332. Choose a two-digit number and multiply its digits together. If the answer you get is another two-digit number, repeat the process of multiplying the digits together until you end up with a single digit. (For example, choosing 48 would require two multiplications, giving you the chain 48 → 32 → 6.) Are there any two-digit numbers that require more than three multiplications to reach a single digit?

Answer, page 250

333. A single set of dominoes has been used to make the "big W" below. However, two halves of two dominoes have been replaced with question marks. The disguised symbols are the black diamond and the single black dot, but not necessarily in that order. Identify the position of each domino.

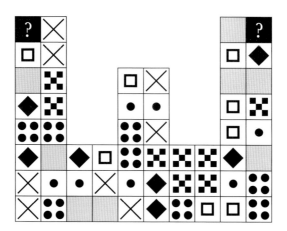

The set of dominoes:

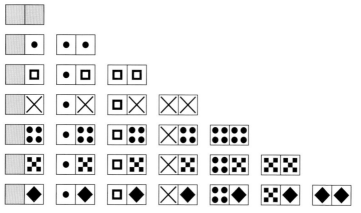

Answer, page 253

334. This puzzle is harder than it looks (and it doesn't look that easy). Find angle BEC.

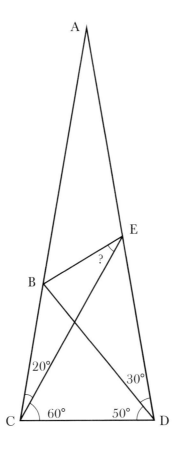

Answer, page 258

335. Take an 8 × 8 chessboard and remove the upper left and bottom right square. Can 31 dominoes, each rectangular and measuring 1 × 2, be placed to cover the chessboard's remaining 62 squares?

Answer, page 257

336. David inherited a rectangular 12-acre plot of land from a great-uncle who lived in the country. Since David prefers the city to the country, he decides to lease out part of the property, but cannot decide how best to subdivide the rectangle or how big the piece he retains should be.

He mentions this to a friend, who offers to divide the property so that it can be broken up into plots of exactly one acre, two acres, three acres, and so on up to twelve acres, to allow David the maximum flexibility in subleasing the land. David is concerned at the cost of doing this, but his friend assures him that it can be done by erecting just two straight fences (which may if necessary cross one another), assuming that adjacent fenced-off plots may be combined when leasing out part of the property.

Where did the friend, who did not know the measurements of the plot of land, suggest the two fences be built?

Answer, page 261

337. A king (who weighs 156 pounds), queen (84 pounds), and prince (72 pounds) are stuck at the top of a tower. A pulley is fixed to the top of the tower, and running over the pulley is a rope with a basket at each end. One basket has a removable 60-pound weight in it. The baskets are only big enough to hold two people or one person and the weight. There are no restrictions on operating the pulley with the baskets empty or with just the weight, but for safety's sake there cannot be more than a 12-pound difference in weight between the two baskets if anyone is in either basket.

How do all three royals escape from the tower?

Answer, page 268

338. What word, expression, or name is depicted below?

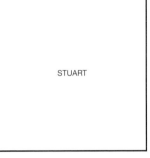

Answer, page 247

339. Arrange the letters below into a 3 × 3 grid to spell six words (three reading across and three reading down).

A E E E H O R S T

Answer, page 255

340. Sixteen tiles, eight black and eight white, have been arranged in a 4 × 4 square as shown. A tile can be moved by picking it up, placing it outside the array at either end of the row or column that it came from, and then closing the gap by sliding that tile (and any tiles between it and the empty space) into the gap to restore the square array.

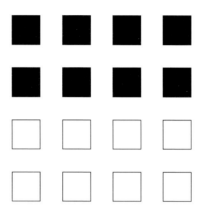

It's easy to find a way of achieving a checkerboard pattern in just eight moves if all the moves are made vertically. Can you find a way to make such a pattern by alternating vertical and horizontal moves?

Answer, page 251

341. A soccer ball consists of a valve, an inner skin, and 32 leather pieces sewn together to make its outer skin. Twenty of these leather pieces are regular hexagons with edges of unit length, and the other twelve are regular pentagons, also with edges of unit length.

If it takes five inches of thread to sew together two unit-length edges of leather, how much thread will be needed to sew the outside skin of the soccer ball?

Answer, page 256

342. What three letters should be placed in the three empty circles so that the longest possible word (which may be more than eight letters long) can be spelled out by reading around the circles? You may start from any circle and read clockwise or counterclockwise.

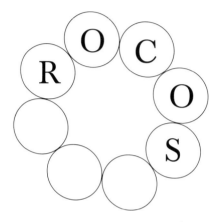

Answer, page 265

343. What type of music is missing below?

___ N B Q K ___ N R

Answer, page 239

344. A traveler in the desert is heading for a camp twelve miles to the north. Five miles to the east of him a road runs in a straight line to the camp. He can travel twice as fast on the road as in the desert. What route should he take to reach the camp in the shortest time?

Answer, page 270

345. You are given four bags of coins; each bag contains thirteen coins. Two of the bags contain genuine coins only, and the other two bags contain counterfeit coins only.

You know the exact weight of a genuine coin, and you also know that counterfeit coins, in comparison to genuine coins, may be one or two grams underweight or overweight.

Counterfeit coins within one bag are all identical to each other, but may or may not be identical to the coins in the other counterfeit bag. How can you identify the two bags of counterfeit coins with a single weighing on a postal scale? (You may take as many coins from as many bags as you like.)

Answer, page 242

346. Three snooker players were presented with an unusual challenge. From a stock of three red and two yellow balls, three balls were chosen at random and each was then concealed in a different box. The challenge was for each player in turn to look inside two of the boxes to see if they could determine the color of the ball in the other box.

The first player looked inside boxes 1 and 3, but was not able to determine the color of the ball in box 2. The second player, having watched player one, then looked inside boxes 2 and 3, but could not then determine the color of the ball in box 1. Having watched players one and two, the third player then stated the color of the ball in one of the boxes, without even bothering to look inside the other two.

Which box did she name, and what was the color of the ball in it?

Answer, page 249

347. A right triangle measuring $5 \times 12 \times 13$ has an area (in square units) equal to its perimeter (in units). Name another right triangle with integral measurements that has this property.

Answer, page 255

348. A, B, C, and D each represent a different word or phrase, and they have a common theme. What are the four words or phrases and what is the theme?

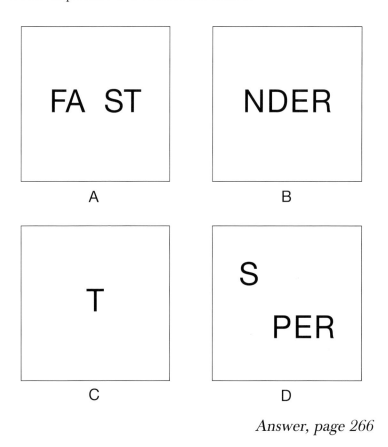

A

B

C

D

Answer, page 266

349. Ten identical squares have been arranged to form the letter E, as shown below:

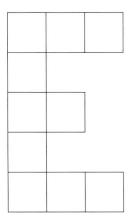

a) Cut the E into five pieces that can then be rearranged to form one large square without flipping over any of the pieces. (Rotating them is allowed, however.)

b) Cut the E into *four* pieces that can then be rearranged to form one large square. This time you are allowed to flip pieces over as well as rotate them.

Answer, page 250

350. In a certain code, the following pairs of words are equal:

acne = made   ahoy = robe   van = bun
fable = flay   pave = ply   beer = yeah

Using this code, what word does "khaki" equal?

Answer, page 259

351. Six people sit down to play a game of Clue, then realize that the board has been mislaid. Undeterred, they agree that each player will simply take turns making a suggestion (or, in due course, an accusation), and that any room can be chosen each time.

A quick refresher on the rules: One character, weapon, and room card are set aside; the rest of the cards are dealt out (with six players, this means everyone will receive three cards). When a suggestion is made, the next player must disprove it if he can; if he holds no cards that match part of the suggestion, the next player must disprove it if he can, and so on.

You are player A, and deal yourself Miss Scarlet, the Revolver, and the Ballroom. The game then progresses with the following suggestions (DB means "disproved by"):

Player	Character	Weapon	Room	DB
B	Col. Mustard	Dagger	Billiard Room	E
C	Prof. Plum	Lead Pipe	Study	E
D	Mrs. White	Wrench	Conservatory	F
E	Mr. Green	Wrench	Library	F
F	Mrs. Peacock	Revolver	Hall	A
A	Mr. Green	Candlestick	Dining Room	F
B	Mrs. Peacock	Rope	Ballroom	E
C	Col. Mustard	Wrench	Lounge	B
D	Prof. Plum	Dagger	Kitchen	B
E	Prof. Plum	Lead Pipe	Study	B
F	Mrs. White	Lead Pipe	Conservatory	E

Player F disproved your suggestion of Mr. Green with the Candlestick in the Dining Room by showing you the Dining Room. Now make the winning accusation.

Answer, page 267

352. Wanda wants to mail a trombone that's 54 inches long at its shortest, but the post office limits parcel sizes to a maximum of 48 inches in length. What can she do?

Answer, page 271

353. Five men are stranded on a desert island whose only other resident is a single monkey. The only food on the island is coconuts. The five men collect all the coconuts they can find, and promise to divide them equally.

The night after they finish collecting the coconuts, the first man (fearing his companions are untrustworthy) decides to take his share while the other castaways are asleep. On dividing the coconuts into five equal piles, he finds there is one coconut left over, so he gives it to the monkey. He then hides his share and puts the rest of the coconuts back into one big pile and goes to sleep.

The second man, unaware that he had been beaten to the punch, then does the same thing. That is, he divides the coconuts into five equal piles, finds one left over that he gives to the monkey, hides what he thinks is his share, and puts the rest back into one big pile. After he goes to sleep, the third, fourth, and fifth men surreptitiously repeat the exercise. So, in all, there were five secret trips that night, and five coconuts for the monkey.

When the sun rose it was obvious to all that many of the coconuts were missing, but, as each man was guilty, none of them said anything about it. Instead, they peacefully divided the remaining coconuts equally, leaving one coconut left over which—you guessed it—they gave to the monkey.

What is the smallest number of coconuts that the fifth man could have ended up with?

Answer, page 253

354. What property having to do with fourth powers do the three numbers below have in common?

1,634   8,208   9,474

355. Samantha, a treasure hunter, found the following message:

From Secret Place to Crossbones Rock
Pace out what steps you may.
Turn right at rock and pace the same
And you'll have found Point A.

Return to Secret Place and count
Your steps to Hangman's Tree.
Turn left at tree and now count down
To take you to point B.

Halfway between points A and B
You'll find my treasure case,
But what a shame that you can't know
About my Secret Place.

She knows where Crossbones Rock and Hangman's Tree are located, but unfortunately does not know the whereabouts of Secret Place. Can you help her find the buried treasure?

356. Find a number between 100,000 and 1,000,000 which is a perfect square and which has its digits in strictly ascending order.

357. Four matches are placed on a table to make a square. Without moving these matches or placing any match on top of another, add four more matches to make three squares in total.

Answer, page 266

358. Here's one for mathematicians. What is the next term in this series?

10   22   36   55   122   220   ?

Answer, page 257

359. How can the five pieces shown below be rearranged (without overlapping) to form a single square?

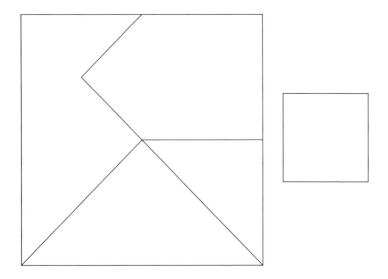

Answer, page 240

360. Andy has several pairs of blue socks and several pairs of gray socks. He keeps them all mixed up in a bag. He tells his aunt what socks he has, and says that if he pulls out two socks at random, there is a 50 percent chance that they will be a matching pair.

Andy's aunt thinks he needs more socks, so she buys him 24 more pairs (some blue, some gray). That's a lot of socks, but Andy's aunt tells him that if he puts these new socks in his bag with the rest, he will still have a 50 percent chance of pulling out a matching pair.

How many socks does Andy now have?

Answer, page 262

361. How many squares are there on a chessboard? (The answer is not 64!)

Answer, page 259

362. Five inventors need to cross a river with their five inventions (one per inventor), using a rowboat that will carry up to three people or inventions in any combination.

The inventors are very secretive about their inventions and each will not allow their invention to be in the presence of another inventor unless they are present too. All of the inventors can row, as can just one of the inventions, which is a robot. The robot, as well as being able to row, can also load and offload itself and any other inventions from the boat.

Before each crossing begins, the boat must be fully emptied before the ship is loaded up again. How can the five inventors cross the river with their inventions, using just the rowboat?

Answer, page 264

363. Here's another puzzle where, given an abbreviated phrase which corresponds to a number (M. in a Y.), the goal is to identify the original phrase (12 = months in a year). Unlike puzzle 315 on page 127, though, here all the abbreviations on a line are equal to each other. On the first line, for instance, 2 (nickels in a dime) = 2 (pints in a quart) = 2 (dice used to play Monopoly).

N. in a D.	=	P. in a Q.	=	D.U. to P.M.
S. in a Y.	=	S. on a S.	=	F. on M.R.
F. in a F.	=	P. on a P.T.	=	C. in S. of an A.
A. on an O.	=	K.H. of E.	=	P. in a G.
P. in a B.A.	=	Y. in a D.	=	L.I.
I. in a F.	=	S. of the Z.	=	D. of C.

Hint: the numbers form a series.

Answer, page 255

364. A five-digit security code is such that in each of the following numbers, one and only one of the digits is in the same position as the security code.

06582	58064
19086	67123
24937	71657
32023	81459
45900	96880

So we can tell from looking at 06582, the first number on the list, that 00000 and 28560 are possible security codes, but 11111 (which has no matches with 06582) and 06999 (which has two matches) are not. What is the security code?

Answer, page 262

365. Near the end of a party, everyone shakes hands with everybody else. Vanessa then arrives and shakes hands with only those people she knows, which is not everyone at the party. By doing this, she increases the total number of handshakes by 25 percent. How many people did Vanessa know?

Answer, page 242

366. A, B, C, and D each represent a different word or phrase, and they have a common theme. What are the four words or phrases and what is the theme?

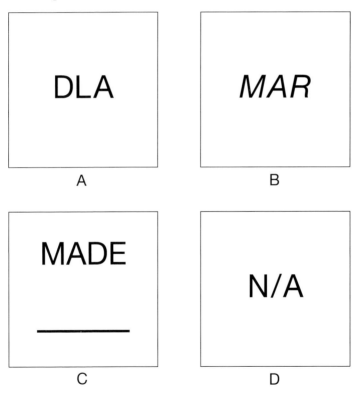

A   B

C   D

Answer, page 250

367. In the diagram below, each of the digits from 1 to 7 inclusive appears exactly eight times. Furthermore, the digits in the eight cells marked with a caret are all the same as each other, as are the digits in the eight cells marked with an asterisk. The sum and product of the digits in each row and column is indicated. Can you reconstruct the grid?

C1	C2	C3	C4	C5	C6	C7	C8	Row totals
		^						Sum: 32 / Product: 24,192
*	*							Sum: 26 / Product: 2,800
								Sum: 13 / Product: 7
^	^	*		^	^			Sum: 26 / Product: 5,670
				*	*			Sum: 26 / Product: 2,800
								Sum: 43 / Product: 326,592
^	^	^		*				Sum: 27 / Product: 7,560
				*	*			Sum: 31 / Product: 22,400

Column totals (left to right):

- Sum: 27 / Product: 4,320
- Sum: 32 / Product: 25,920
- Sum: 32 / Product: 8,640
- Sum: 28 / Product: 5,764,801
- Sum: 56 / Product: 384
- Sum: 19 / Product: 13,500
- Sum: 32 / Product: 14,400
- Sum: 30 / Product: 14,400

Once you've done that, give yourself a brief pat on the back and then take a deep breath: the puzzle's not finished quite yet! You see, the diagram was originally constructed from the 28 domino pieces shown on the top of the next page:

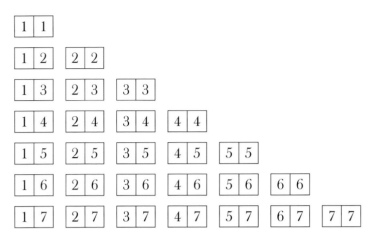

To complete the puzzle, reconstruct the original grid by placing all the dominoes in the correct location.

Answer, page 239

368. A Pythagorean triangle has an area of 666,666. No side of this triangle shares a common factor with another side or is smaller than 666. What is the length of the triangle's hypotenuse?

Answer, page 269

369. In 1998, the U.K. Institute of Actuaries celebrated its 150th anniversary. At that time, a puzzle was proposed that asked for each of the integers from 1 to 150 to be made using only the digits 1, 9, 9, and 8; parentheses as required; and the standard mathematical symbols: $+$, $-$, $\times$, $\div$, $\sqrt{}$, ! (factorial), decimal point, and $^-$ (repeating decimal).

The number that eluded most would-be solvers was 148. It isn't easy to find, but there is a solution for this number as well. What is it?

Answer, page 266

370. An orienteer climbs two hills, A and B, and on the top of each measures the angle between a familiar landmark and the top of the other hill. Having done this, she notices that one angle is twice the other. Checking her map, she then sees that A and B are five miles apart, and that the distances between the hilltops and the landmark are four and six miles as shown:

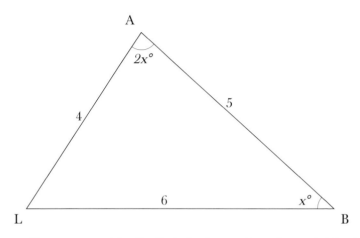

Prove geometrically that she has not made a mistake in her measurements.

Answer, page 244

371. A teacher wrote the number 139,257 on the blackboard and asked the class to write the number in base 8. One student noticed that the answer, 417,771, is three times the first number if both numbers are considered to be in base 10.

What are the lowest and highest numbers (in base 10) to have this property?

Answer, page 241

372. Tom, Dick, and Harry met for a picnic. Tom brought 15 items, Dick brought 9 items, and Harry brought 8 coins of equal value to be shared by the other two as a reimbursement for bringing food for him to share.

Assuming the men consumed equal shares of food (and all the items are of equal value), how should the money be divided?

Answer, page 246

373. What is the smallest right triangle that will completely fit inside another right triangle for which:

- The larger triangle has a side that is shorter than all three of the smaller triangle's sides.
- All six sides are integral.

Answer, page 262

374. There is a well-known person whose name, when entered into the second and fourth rows of the diagram below, will spell five-letter words in all seven columns. Who is it?

C	A	W	C	C	S	A
B	R	O	T	A	D	E
E	M	G	H	S	Y	D

Answer, page 251

375. Using the digits 1 to 9 in ascending order, a standard arithmetical sign between each pair of digits, and parentheses as required, find an alternative expression to the one below that still equals 100.

$$1 + 2 + 3 + 4 + 5 + 6 + 7 + (8 \times 9) = 100$$

Answer, page 256

376. In the game of bridge, hands are commonly assessed by assigning points to the high cards using the system below, and then adding up the points:

- 4 points for an ace
- 3 points for a king
- 2 points for a queen
- 1 point for a jack

Can you find a distribution of cards in which a partnership can make a grand slam against any defense, but with the partnership having the smallest possible number of points?

Answer, page 241

377. A $3 \times 3 \times 3$ magic cube is a cube made of 27 smaller cubes (numbered from 1 to 27) where all the rows, columns, pillars, and main diagonals (the ones that pass through the center of the cube) have a common sum.

Is it possible to find such a $3 \times 3 \times 3$ magic cube where the central cube is numbered 14? What about a $3 \times 3 \times 3$ magic cube where the central cube is *not* numbered 14?

Answer, page 263

378. The diagram below shows an arrangement of the ten digits from 0 to 9 in ten circles, where the sums formed by adding the numbers in each pair of adjacent circles are all different.

If you rearrange the ten digits in the circles, what is the smallest number of different sums for adjacent circles that can be achieved?

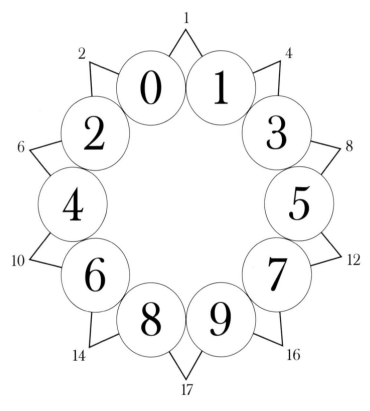

Answer, page 265

379. Can you rearrange the seven letters in the phrase NEW DOOR to spell one word?

Answer, page 248

380. The number 120 has the property that the sum of its divisors (1, 2, 3, 4, 5, 6, 8, 10, 12, 15, 20, 24, 30, 40, 60, and 120) is equal to three times the original number. What other three-digit number has divisors that sum to exactly three times the original number?

Answer, page 266

381. In the expression below, each letter represents a different digit from 1 to 9.

$$\frac{A}{DE} \;+\; \frac{B}{FG} \;+\; \frac{C}{HI} \;=\; 1$$

What are the three fractions?

Answer, page 253

382. Using the digits 1, 2, 3, 4, and 5 exactly once each in each expression, parentheses, decimal points (but not repeating decimals), and the standard arithmetical symbols +, −, ×, and ÷, find expressions equal to 111, 222, 333, 444, 555, 666, 777, 888, and 999.

Answer, page 240

383. Almost all whole numbers can be expressed as the sum of no more than eight positive cubes. For example, the number 121 needs only six:

$$121 = 4^3 + 3^3 + 3^3 + 1^3 + 1^3 + 1^3$$

Remarkably, there are just two exceptions to this rule. The first is 23, which needs nine positive cubes $(2^3 + 2^3 + 1^3 + 1^3 + 1^3 + 1^3 + 1^3 + 1^3 + 1^3)$, and the second is 239, which also needs nine positive cubes, but which can be solved in two different ways. What are they?

Answer, page 256

384. A set of dominoes, plus one extra double (a duplicate of one of the double dominoes in the set), was used to make the shape below. The symbol on the extra double also appears in the upper left and upper right corners of the shape, but has been replaced with question marks. Can you identify the position of each domino?

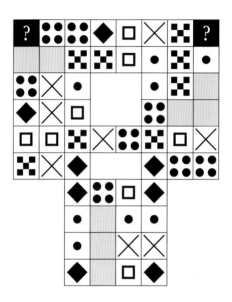

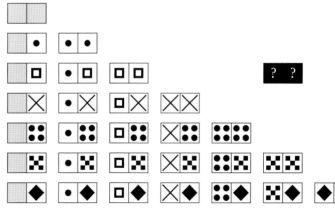

Answer, page 243

385. Fill in the empty squares in the grid below according to the following rules:

- Each square must contain one of the digits from 1 to 7.
- In each of the four rows and four columns, each of the digits from 1 to 7 must appear exactly once.
- Each of the white numbers already contained within the grid must equal the sum of the eight digits surrounding it.

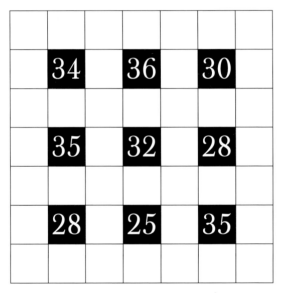

Answer, page 268

386. Here's another one for mathematicians. What is the next term in this series?

2   12   36   80   150   ?

Answer, page 247

387. What word, expression, or name is depicted below?

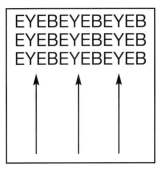

Answer, page 251

388. Which word is the odd one out?

laughing   canopy   stupid
understudy   hijack   burst

Answer, page 265

389. The military base of a fighting unit has four missiles to protect it from attack by air. The missiles are placed 50 miles north, 50 miles east, 50 miles south, and 50 miles west of the military base. Each missile has a range of 70 miles and is designed to harmlessly self-destruct if it does not hit its target before reaching the end of its range.

During a training exercise in which each missile was pointing to the next missile clockwise around the base, the four missiles were accidentally and simultaneously fired, sending them on a spiral route centered on the base. If the missiles collide above the base, then the base will be destroyed. Will the missiles get that far, or will the base survive?

Answer, page 245

390. Without using trial and error, find the number n and the digit d in the following equation:

$$[3 \times (300 + n)]^2 = 898{,}d04$$

Answer, page 271

391. An astronaut, hoping to discover life on the moon, laid a trip wire around the moon's equator that was just two inches clear of the surface. He didn't catch anything, so he decided to raise the wire to six inches above the surface. The moon has a diameter of 2,160 miles. How much extra wire will he need? (Assume the moon is perfectly spherical.)

Answer, page 257

392. A car is parked on a steep hill when the brakes suddenly fail. In the first second, the car rolls 12 inches. How far will it have rolled after five seconds?

Answer, page 244

393. In the multiplication problem below, each of the digits from 0 to 9 occurs exactly twice.

$$
\begin{array}{r}
\text{\_ \_ \_} \\
\times \ \underline{\text{\_ \_ \_}} \\
\text{\_ \_ \_} \\
\text{\_ \_ \_} \\
\underline{\text{\_ \_ \_}} \\
\text{\_ \_ \_ \_ \_}
\end{array}
$$

Can you reconstruct the problem?

Answer, page 243

394. Find a ten-digit number where the last ten digits of its square equal the original ten-digit number. An example using three digits is 376, the square of which is 141,376.

Answer, page 248

395. Just by guessing (and using some inspiration!), can you find the square root of this number?

$$12,345,678,987,654,321$$

Answer, page 253

396. Each empty square in the grid below is to be filled with a single letter. When read consecutively (inserting spaces where appropriate), the 18 letters spell out a well-known object.

The numbers in the grid represent the difference in value between adjacent letters, when each letter is given a numerical value equal to its position in the alphabet (that is, A = 1, B = 2, C = 3, and so on up to Z = 26). So, the digit 4 in the grid could separate the letters A and E, B and F, C and G, and so on. What is the object?

	7		4		13		5		5	
5	■	15	■	14	■	9	■	4	■	4
	13		5		8		18		13	
8	■	14	■	1	■	14	■	14	■	17
	9		10		7		10		18	

Answer, page 250

397. Without rotating any of the 16 pieces in the square below, rearrange them to make another square with common eight-letter names reading across each row.

Hint: The names alternate between male and female.

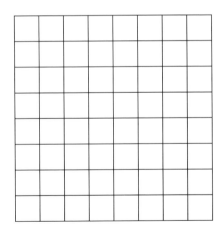

Answer, page 266

398. I'm thinking of four positive integers that are different from each other, and that total less than 18. If I told you both their product and the smallest of the four integers, you'd be able to identify all four numbers. But you don't know their product and you don't know the smallest integer . . . or do you?

Answer, page 260

399. Is it true that the capital of Norway is in Czechoslovakia?

Answer, page 269

400. If TED^3 = VINDICATE, and different letters represent different digits, is it DAVE or VIC that is two times IAN?

Answer, page 241

401. The name of a famous 20th-century world leader is depicted below. Who is it?

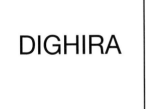

Answer, page 267

402. Would it be easier for a helicopter to take off from the surface of the moon or the surface of the earth?

Answer, page 255

403. What is the next term in this series?

A E F H I K ?

Answer, page 238

404. The diagram below shows two circuits. The top circuit contains two 1-ohm resistors in series and has a resistance of 2 ohms. The bottom circuit contains two 1-ohm resistors in parallel and has a resistance of 0.5 ohms.

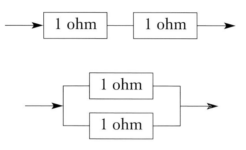

The circuit below is also composed of 1-ohm resistors. What is the resistance of the circuit?

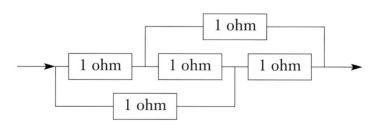

Answer, page 251

405. The variables a, b, and c represent three different nonzero digits. Find their values, given that the three-digit number $abc = b^c - a$.

Answer, page 271

406. Garfath Crescent is a semicircle whose diameter is an exact number of yards and less than a mile (1,760 yards). Along its straight side runs a hedge, and on its curved side stand 26 trees. (The diagram does not show their placement to scale.)

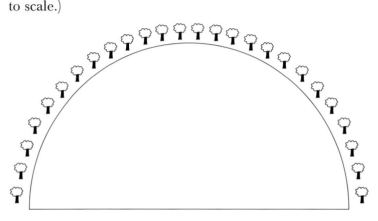

The distance from the center of any tree to either end of the hedge is a nonzero, integral number of yards. How long is the hedge?

Answer, page 246

407. An incomplete ten-digit code (using all the digits from 0 to 9) is shown below. It's an easy code to remember, as it is based on a particular well-known pattern. Are the two digits in the middle 17 or 71?

8 5 4 9 ? ? 6 3 2 0

Answer, page 257

408. A man-made pond has a flat base and vertical sides. In the center of the pond, a statue is to be erected using three identical concrete cubes (placed side by side) as the statue's foundation.

When the first concrete cube is placed flat on the bottom of the pond, the water level rises three inches. When the second and third concrete cubes are placed flat on the bottom of the pond, the water level rises four inches on both occasions. How big are the cubes?

Answer, page 252

409. What word, expression, or name is depicted below?

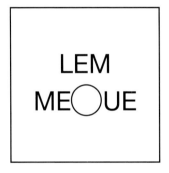

Answer, page 241

410. A man decreed in his will that $240,000 should be divided equally among his grandchildren—but only those who were monks or nuns at the time of his death. When he died, the monks received the same total amount as the nuns, and each of the grandchildren who benefited from his bequest received $56,000 more than they would have if all of the man's grandchildren had shared the money equally.

How many grandchildren did the man have when he died?

Answer, page 249

411. The winner of a game show is offered a choice of three envelopes, one of which contains a check for a million dollars while the other two contain small gift certificates. The contestant knows the contents of the envelopes, but doesn't know which one contains the grand prize.

Once the contestant has chosen an envelope, the game show host (who does know the contents of each envelope) then opens one of the remaining two envelopes to reveal a gift certificate, as he always does. He then asks the contestant if he wants to keep the envelope he has already chosen or swap it for the remaining unopened one.

What should the contestant do, and what is his chance of winning the grand prize?

Answer, page 243

412. Wht s th lwst whl nmbr tht wld nt b dscrbd nql f t wr wrttn n th sm stl s ths qstn?

Answer, page 266

413. The finals of the Tiddlywinks Club Championship features two players: Tiddle and Wink. Both players know that in any one game between them, Tiddle's chance of winning is two in three.

The championship is a best-of-nine series. Tiddle says that, according to the odds, after six games the score should be 4–2 to him, but to save time, he'd be willing to start the championship from a base score of 3–2 in his favor, thereby leaving Wink a chance of being tied 3–3 after game six.

Wink would like to give himself the best chance of winning the championship. Should he accept Tiddle's offer?

Answer, page 264

414. Susie swims at a constant speed. The distance from the jetty to where her boat is moored would normally take Susie ten minutes to swim. However, because she has the current with her, she is able to swim from the jetty to her boat in exactly five minutes. How long will it take her to swim back?

Answer, page 259

415. I bought four items from my local convenience store. The bill came to $7.11. I thought that amount must have been wrong, as I had seen the cashier multiplying the four prices together instead of adding them. (The cash register was broken, so he had to use a calculator instead.)

When I questioned the cashier about it, he agreed that he had multiplied the prices together, but said that in this case it didn't matter since the sum of the four items was also $7.11.

What were the prices of the four items?

Answer, page 262

416. What piece of equipment used more in New York than in Florida is depicted below?

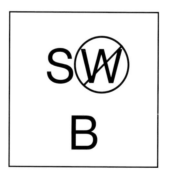

Answer, page 245

417. A triangular farm is divided into four paddocks by fences that run in straight lines from two of the corners as shown below:

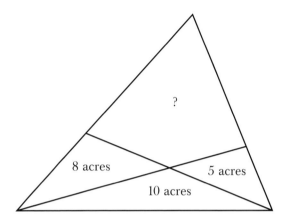

The areas of the three triangular paddocks are as shown. What is the area of the other paddock?

Answer, page 238

418. Two friends, Alvin and Brendan, played a 25-game tournament of horseshoes one day. They agreed that, to decide the winner of the tournament, instead of counting the number of games each player won, they would count the overall number of points scored.

Alvin started the first game, and after that, the player to throw first was the person who won the previous game. (None of the games were tied.) Over the course of the 25 games, Alvin won six of the games in which he threw first, and Brendan won seven of the games in which he threw first.

After 24 games, Alvin and Brendan had each scored the same number of points. Which player won the 25th game and therefore the tournament?

Answer, page 268

419. You are a contestant on a game show on which you have been presented with the following challenge.

You are put in a booth from which you cannot see out, but the audience can see in. There are three identical switches in front of you; there is nothing else in the booth. Two of the switches work clear light bulbs displayed on a stand on the main stage of the studio; the third works a green bulb on the same stand. All of the switches are in the "off" position when you enter the booth.

After you have flipped whichever switches you decide to flip, you will have to leave the booth to see which bulbs are lit. Once you have left the booth, you will not be allowed to reenter it. Your challenge is to determine which switch controls the green bulb, and you have two minutes to do so.

Of course, you could just guess which switch controls the green bulb, which would give you a one in three chance of winning the challenge. But there is a way to be 100 percent certain that you will win. What is it?

Answer, page 240

420. What word, expression, or name is depicted below?

Ms. Paprika
Miss Rosemary
Madame Sage
Mrs. Oregano

Answer, page 260

ANSWERS

88.

Position	Team	Captain	Color
1	United	Cooke	Red
2	Rovers	Allen	Blue
3	County	Dixon	White
4	Albion	Evans	Yellow
5	Thistle	Boyle	Green

154. Of all possible sets of four whole numbers whose product is 180, the only sets with sums that are not unique are those with sums of 18 and 22. Thus the professor must have been teaching for one of those two periods.

If it is 18 years, then the four lengths of study could be 1, 5, 6, and 6 years; 2, 2, 5, and 9 years; or 2, 3, 3, and 10 years. If it is 22 years, then the possible combinations are 1, 2, 9, and 10 years, or 2, 2, 3, and 15 years.

We are told that knowing whether any of the students were into double figures would enable the professor to determine the four periods, so a length of teaching of 22 years is ruled out. Of the three sets whose sum is 18 years, two contain no double-digit numbers, which leaves the third set as the only possibility.

Thus the four students had been studying for 2, 3, 3, and 10 years.

91. Forgive and forget.

28. ANGST, ABYSS, BAWDY, COMFY, DENIM, EXPEL, FAKIR, MAJOR, PIQUE, SERVE, TITLE, TOPAZ, WINCH.

102. The verse asks whether $10^{1/10} > 2^{1/3}$ or, if we raise each side to the power of 30, whether $10^3 > 2^{10}$? The answer is "no."

62. Five across is three factorial, which is SIX. Two-thirds of SIX or, more precisely, the last two-thirds of the word SIX, is IX, which is the Roman numeral nine.

106. By crossing out "SIX LETTERS," we are left with the word "BANANA."

18. Smith served first. One possible proof is as follows:

Whoever served first would have served on 20 of the points played and the other player would have served on 17 of them. Suppose the first player won x of the points on which he served and y of the points served by his opponent. The total number of points lost by the player who served them is then 20 − x + y. This must equal 13, since we are told that 24 of the 37 points were won by the player serving. Thus x = 7 + y, and the first server won (7 + y) + y = 7 + 2y points in total. This is an odd number, and only Smith won an odd number of points. Thus Smith served first.

27. Mixed bag.

92. 50,123 − 49,876 = 247.

75. ♠2, ♥9, ♥5, ♦4, ♣8.

2. 3,816,547,290.

21. The envelope with the formula is Envelope 3.

54. The maximum number of blocks in the set is 55.

If only three of the five available colors are used, then opposite faces of a block must have the same color. Thus by symmetry there is only one way in which a block can be painted with any three given colors, and there are ten different ways in which three colors can be chosen.

If four colors are used, then two pairs of opposite faces must each have the same color. By symmetry it doesn't matter which way around the other two faces are painted. The colors for the two pairs of matching faces can be chosen in ten different ways, and the other two colors can then be chosen in three ways, giving an overall total of 30 combinations.

Finally, if five colors are used then just one pair of opposite faces will have the same color. The remaining four colors can be arranged in three different ways, so using five colors gives a total of $5 \times 3 = 15$ combinations.

The maximum number of blocks in the set is therefore $10 + 30 + 15 = 55$.

19. White's key move of **1** Ka5!! seems self-destructive and a sure provocation for Black to play **1** ... e1(Q)+. White's reply, **2** Kb6!, seems even more provocative as it offers Black no fewer than seven different moves with which to check White's king. Each one, however, can be defended by moving the knight at c6 for a discovered checkmate. If Black moves **1** ... Rg7 then **2** Ne7+ Ka7 **3** Nc8 mate. If **1** ... Rg5 then **2** Kb6 (threatening **3** Ne7 mate) Rxd5 **3** Nc7 mate. If **1** ... Kb7 then **2** Ne7+ Ka7 **3** Nc8 mate.

132. The letters are the first letters of the words in the question. Thus the next two letters are A and W.

151. ABCDE is 93084.

5. $\sqrt{.2^{-2}}$, which shows that two 2's can make five!

112. Long underwear.

78. On the double.

11. AAKAAKKK.

3. Eleven students passed Exam One only, three passed Exam Two only, and eight passed Exam Three only. Thus ten students passed more than one exam.

98. Regrouping the sequence as 20, 21, 22, 23, 24, 25, 26, 27, 28, it is obvious the next three terms in this more normal format are 29, 30, and 31. Using the question's format, the required answer is 293 and 031.

135.

```
        7   7   5
            3   3
      ─────────────
    2   3   2   5
2   3   2   5
─────────────────
2   5   5   7   5
```

23. The series is generated by counting the number of characters in the corresponding Roman numeral, as shown for the first ten numbers below:

I	II	III	IV	V	VI	VII	VIII	IX	X
1	2	3	2	1	2	3	4	2	1

The first term to equal 10 is the 288th in the series: CCLXXXVIII. Thus the answer to the question is Brutus.

145. *Little House on the Prairie.*

143. 6174.

55. There are 26 former committee members (9 of whom are women), 27 committee members, and 39 members who have never been on the committee. This gives a total of 92 members.

96. To prove this, color the large triangle of 36 units in area as shown, giving 21 light and 15 dark unit triangles.

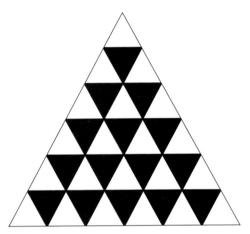

If the twelve available shapes are colored in a similar manner, ten are found to have an equal number of light and dark unit triangles. In the remaining two cases, there are four light and two dark (or vice versa). However, to tile the shape above requires at least three pieces where the difference between the numbers of light and dark triangles is two. Since there are only two such pieces, no solution is possible.

165. My father was born in 1927 $(2^{11} - 11^2)$, and his grandfather in 1844 $(3^7 - 7^3)$.

126. In the diagram below, the two smaller triangles are similar, which means the ratio of their sides is constant and more particularly, that $y/1 = 1/x$.

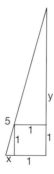

By the Pythagorean theorem
$(x + 1)^2 + (y + 1)^2 = (x + 1)^2 + (1/x + 1)^2 = 25$ so
$x^4 + 2x^3 + 2x^2 + 2x + 1 = 25x^2$ from which
$(x^2 + x + 1)^2 = 26x^2$ so
$x^2 + (1 - \sqrt{26})x + 1 = 0$ and $x = 0.2605$ meters.

The base of the ladder is 1.2605 meters from the wall.

8. No U-Turn.

59. Cornerstone.

164. The number at the center of any 3×3 magic square is always one-third of the magic square's constant. Thus the center square must be 37. The rest then follows. (Reflected and rotated answers are also possible.)

43	1	67
61	37	13
7	73	31

30. Either 1, 2, 6, 7, 9, 14, 15, 18, 20 or 1, 3, 6, 7, 12, 14, 15, 19, 20.

7. For White to win, he has to force one of Black's knights to move. Then, provided White's king is safe from unwanted checks and White has not moved his own knights, White wins with Ne4 mate or Nd5 mate. The actual winning move will depend upon which knight Black eventually moves.

Black can delay moving a knight for 59 moves! His tactic is to shunt the rook at a4 to and fro to a3 whenever he can. Accordingly, and taking the route that avoids unwanted checks, White uses his king to inhibit the shunting rook by timing the arrival of his king at b5 to follow Black's move Ra3.

On the first four occasions White does this, Black keeps his rook out of danger by moving a pawn on the e file. On the fifth occasion, to avoid moving a knight and to save his rook, Black must block his rook in with a5-a4. On his next move Black is compelled to move a knight and expose himself to an instant checkmate. Note that if Black moves his pawns before he has to, then the mate is simply speeded up. With Black's best defense as shown below, White will mate in sixty.

White's first move can be either Ke8 or Kd6. White's king then proceeds d7, c8, b7, b6, b5. By moving to d7 via e8 or d6, the White king arrives at b5 after an even number of moves. Thus, for move six, Black's shunting rook will be at a3 and Black must move a pawn, lose his rook, or be mated. To defer mate as long as possible, Black must play e4-e3.

After Black's move, e4-e3, White moves his king away from b5 and Black can continue with the shunting of his rook. White must now move his king back to b5 in an odd number of moves in order to catch the shunting rook at a3. The shortest route for White to achieve this that avoids unwanted checks is b6, b7, c8, d7, e8, f8, f7, e8, d7, c8, b7, b6, b5, and this he repeats four times.

On moves 19, 32, and 45 Black takes a break from shunting his rook and moves a pawn on the e file. On move 58, however, Black can do no better than to block his rook in with a5-a4. White then plays a waiting move, Kb6. If Black moves the knight at b4, then White mates with Nd5, and if Black moves the knight at d2, then White mates with Ne4. This gives White mate in sixty.

104. Back and forth.

131. The terms in the series are 100 in base 10, 100 in base 9, 100 in base 8, …, 100 in base 5. The next term in the series is 100 in base 4, which is 1210.

58. Regrouping the series as 1, 2, 4, 8, 16, 32, 64, 128, and 256, the next two terms in this series are 512 and 1024. The answer to the question is 5121.

42. Supplements to use are: 8, 12, 14, 17, 18, 19, 20, 21, 22, 23, 25, 26, 27, 29, 30, 31, 33, 35, 37, 39, 41, 43, 45, 47, and 49. They total 711.

120. Safety in numbers.

52. Not eleven, but ten times. The times are between 1 and 2, between 2 and 3, and so on, ending with once between 10 and 11. It does not happen between 11 and 12, since it happens at exactly 12 (noon and midnight). The question excludes noon and midnight, so that occurrence doesn't count.

81. $96,420 \times 87,531 = 8,439,739,020$.

1. Red in the face.

110. Let the radius of the largest ball that will fit in the gap be r, and let the distance from the corner to the center of the smaller ball be y.

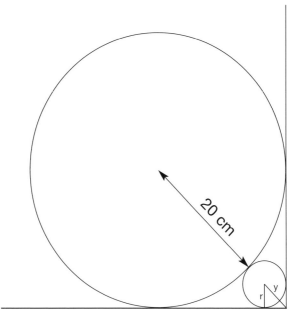

The distance from the corner to the center of the big ball is $20 + r + y = \sqrt{(20^2 + 20^2)}$, so $r + y = \sqrt{800} - 20 = 8.28$ cm. Since $y = \sqrt{(r^2 + r^2)}$, $2r^2 = (8.28 - r)^2$, from which $r^2 + 16.57r - 68.63 = 0$ and $r = 3.43$ cm. This means that the largest ball that can fit in the gap has diameter $2 \times 3.43 = 6.86$ cm, so the answer to the original question is no.

121. $3^{1/8} \times 3^{1/5} = 2^{5/8} \times {}^{16}/_5 = 10.$

$3 \times \sqrt[3]{37} = \sqrt[3]{(27 \times 37)} = \sqrt[3]{999} < \sqrt[3]{1000} = 10.$

160. Monday is an anagram of dynamo.

35. At the point of no return.

45. Each line describes the line above. For example, since line five is 1 1 1 2 2 1, which can be expressed as three ones (3 1), two twos (2 2), and one one (1 1), line six is 3 1 2 2 1 1.

The tenth line in the pyramid is therefore:

1 3 2 1 1 3 1 1 1 2 3 1 1 3 1 1 2 2 1 1

38. Pin-up.

20. Forever and ever.

157. The positions were first, fifth, and ninth for the navy; second, sixth, and seventh for the air force; and third, fourth, and eighth for the army.

103.

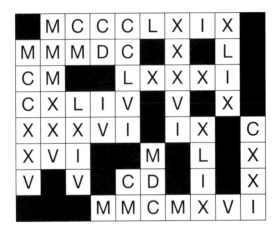

111. Count Dracula.

17. Ambiguous.

56. The series consists of the numbers of letters in the words one, two, three, etc.

122. Rewriting each ANNE in base 10, we have:

$$A(8^3 - 5^3 - 7^3) + N(8^2 + 8 - 5^2 - 5 - 7^2 - 7) + E(1 - 1 - 1) = 0$$

That is, $44A - 14N - E = 0$. Noting that A, N, and E are all digits of a number written in base 5, so A, N, and E are all less than five, $A = 1$, $N = 3$, and $E = 2$ is the unique solution. Thus the three letters do represent three different digits.

40. F for February. The letters are the initials of the first eight months of the year.

152. The key move is **1** Bh3, to which Black must reply with a queen move. If Black plays **1** ... Qa8 or **1** ... Qe8, then **2** Qd4+ Qe4 **3** Qf6+ Qf5 **4** Qg5+ Qxg5 mate.

If Black keeps his queen on the same rank, say **1** ... Qd4, then **2** g3+ Kf3+ **3** Bg4+ Qxg4 mate.

If Black plays any other queen move, then White plays either **2** Qb4+ or **2** Qc4+ or **2** Qd4+ forcing Black to reply with either **2** ... Qxb4 or **2** ... Qxc4 or **2** ... Qxd4 and then White forces Black to win as above. For example, **1** Bh3 Qa6 **2** Qc4+ Qxc4 **3** g3+ Kf3+ **4** Bg4+ Qxg4 mate.

82. Income tax.

43. The solutions are 1,872,549,630 and 7,812,549,630, and are derived as follows: The 5 and 0 can be placed immediately. The sixth digit must be 4. The seventh digit is odd (since every second digit must be even), so it must be 9. The eighth digit must be 6. The ninth digit must be 3. The third digit is 1 or 7, so the fourth digit must be 2. The first three digits are therefore 187 or 781.

66. Split-second timing.

105. Let the radii of the larger and smaller circles be R and r respectively. The desired area is then $\pi R^2 - \pi r^2 = \pi(R^2 - r^2)$.

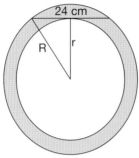

Using the Pythagorean theorem, it can be seen that $R^2 - r^2 = (^{24}/_2)^2 = 144$, so the desired area is $144\pi = 452.4$ sq. cm.

39. The value of 1,997 nickels is $99.85, 25 cents more than 1,992 nickels (worth $99.60).

125. Black's last move was a7-a5. It could not have been a6-a5 since a pawn at a6 would have had to capture White's pawn. Neither could it have been b6xa5 since this would imply, given the position of Black's other pawns, that Black had made nine captures (which is impossible since White still has eight pieces on the board). Thus White plays **1** bxa6 e.p.

White wins by being stalemated as follows: **1** ... bxa6 **2** b5 axb5 **3** f5 any, and White is stalemated.

51. 8128.

71. $4! + 5! + 7! = 24 + 120 + 5040 = (5^2 - 1) + (11^2 - 1) + (71^2 - 1) = 72^2$.

108. $325 = 1^2 + 18^2 = 6^2 + 17^2 = 10^2 + 15^2$.

34. White marbles can only be removed from the box in pairs. There is an odd number of white marbles to start with, so the last marble in the box will be white.

90. Other than rotations and reflections there is only one solution. The best way to start is with the central number, which must be a factor of 45, the sum of all nine numbers.

5	1	4
6	3	8
2	7	9

63. Anyone for tennis?

65. The players scored 5, 7, 11, 13, 17, 19, 29, 31, 37, 41, and 43 goals. Their average was 23 goals.

149. $71 = (4! + 4.4) / .4$

47. $21978 \times 4 = 87912$

77. Sweet tooth.

129. Out of court.

139. 1 Qe6+ Kh8 **2** Nf7+ Kg8 **3** Nh6+ Kh8 **4** Qg8+ Rxg8 **5** Nf7 mate.

153. Bob up and down.

87. 4 and 3. The numbers are the numbers of letters in the words of the question.

24. To show the perimeter is divided into two equal lengths, whatever the angle of the arrow, let the diameter of each of the smaller semicircles (and thus the radius of the large semicircle) be d and let the arrow lie at an angle of a radians to the horizontal.

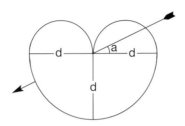

The perimeter length lying above the horizontal line is $\pi d/2 + \pi d/2 = \pi d$, which is the perimeter length lying below the horizontal line. Therefore, to prove the heart's perimeter is divided into two equal lengths, we need to show that the part of the perimeter above the horizontal line and below the arrow is equal in length to the part of the perimeter that is below the horizontal line and above the arrow.

Begin by letting C be the center of the smaller semicircle on the right as shown below:

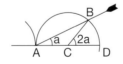

Since triangle ABC is isosceles, angle BCD is 2a radians. Thus the length of arc BD is $^{2a}/_{2\pi}$ multiplied by the perimeter of the small circle $= {}^{2a}/_{2\pi} \times \pi d = ad$. This is also the length of the arc of the big semicircle that is below the horizontal line and above the arrow and so the result is proven.

156. Lucky break.

60. Old is 30 and Young is 18.

107. Weeping willow.

101. Maverick, subtle (or bustle), pique, golfer, jinx, wrap, brazen, and holiday.

118. 3,782,915,460.

146. The pairs are:

$$^{355}/_{113} = 3.1415929... \quad (\pi = 3.1415926...)$$
$$^{577}/_{408} = 1.414215... \quad (\sqrt{2} = 1.414213...)$$
$$^{878}/_{323} = 2.71826... \quad (e = 2.71828...)$$
$$^{987}/_{610} = 1.618032... \quad (\phi = 1.618033...)$$

where π is the area of a circle of unit radius, e is the base for natural logarithms, and ϕ is the golden ratio. Interesting properties of ϕ include its relationship with its square (which equals $\phi + 1$) and its reciprocal (which equals $\phi - 1$). $\phi = (1 + \sqrt{5}) / 2$.

137. 916.

44. One step forward, two steps back.

83. The diagram contains 47 triangles in total, as below:

1 triangle of full size   6 triangles of $^1/_2$ size
3 triangles of $^1/_3$ size   10 triangles of $^1/_4$ size
6 triangles of $^1/_6$ size   12 triangles of $^1/_8$ size
3 triangles of $^1/_{12}$ size   6 triangles of $^1/_{24}$ size

13. Round of drinks on the house.

46. Reading between the lines.

161. The hands on the clock face show roughly when Heather left her room. The hour hand has moved $(x - 35)$ minutes since 7 P.M., and the minute hand y minutes. Since the minute hand moves twelve times faster than the hour hand, $y = 12(x - 35)$.

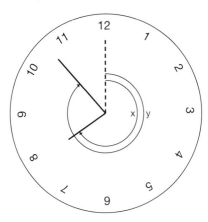

Now consider the position when the hands have changed places. The hour hand will have moved $(y - 50)$ minutes since 10 P.M., and the minute hand x minutes. Hence $x = 12(y - 50)$.

Solving these equations, $x = 39^{63}/_{143}$ and $y = 53^{41}/_{143}$. Thus the time elapsed since Heather left her room was 2 hours 46 minutes $9^{3}/_{13}$ seconds.

150. "We" are the number of letters in each word. Thus "twelve" is six, "nine" is four, etc.

113. 1 bxa8(N) Kxg2 **2** Nb6 any **3** a8(B or Q) mate. Note that White's second move prevents **2** ... Bxa7.

138. The three names are Arnold, Roland, and Ronald.

9. 2,100,010,006.

166. Robin Hood.

133. Construct another regular five-pointed star as shown in the diagram. Since both are regular stars, $^{AB}/_{BC} = {}^{AD}/_{DB}$.

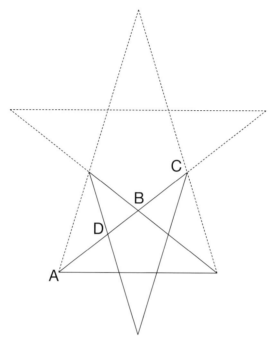

Let AB be of unit length and AD = BC = x (so DB = 1 − x). Then: $^{AB}/_{BC} = {}^{AD}/_{DB}$ so $^{1}/_{x} = {}^{x}/_{(1-x)}$.

So $x^2 + x − 1 = 0$, $x = −^{1}/_{2} + {}^{1}/_{2}\sqrt{5} = 0.618034$, and the ratio of AB to BC is the reciprocal of 0.618034, which is 1.618034.

41. A won against B, C, and D with scores of 3-0, 1-0, and 2-1 respectively. B won against C with a score of 1-0 and tied D with a score of 1-1. C won against D with a score of 2-0.

159. 1 d4 d5 **2** Qd3 Qd6 **3** Qh3 Qh6 **4** Qxc8 mate.

67. Despite being the worst shot of the three, Arthur has the best chance of surviving, with a probability of .5222. Allwyn has the next best chance of surviving at .3 and Aitkins the least chance at .1778.

Arthur's tactic will be to aim to miss if the other two are alive. This is because the other two, if they get the choice, will fire at each other rather than Arthur. This will leave Arthur with the first shot at the survivor. The reason that Allwyn would choose to fire at Aitkins rather than Arthur is that he would rather have Arthur shooting at him with a 50% hit rate than Aitkins with an 80% success rate. The decision for Aitkins to fire at Allwyn rather than Arthur, if he gets the choice, is because for Aitkins to fire successfully at Arthur would be to sign his own death warrant.

72. By factorizing 2,450 and then compiling a list of the age groups with the desired product, it is found that only two have the same sum, namely 64. Thus Jim is 32, and the three passengers are either 50, 7, and 7 or 49, 10, and 5.

When he was told there was someone older than Bob on the bus, Jim was able to determine the passengers' ages. Obviously Bob cannot be older than 49, and if he were younger than this then both groups would still have been acceptable. Thus, knowing Bob was 49, Jim was able to determine the three passengers were aged 50, 7, and 7.

93. If this position had occurred in a real game, then Black's last move must have been g7-g5. Therefore, White can force mate in two with 1 hxg6 e.p. Kh5 2 Rxh7 mate.

85. Receding hairline.

86.

```
            6   6 . 3   7   5
1   6 ) 1   0   6   2
            9   6
            1   0   2
                9   6
                    6   0
                    4   8
                    1   2   0
                    1   1   2
                            8   0
                            8   0
```

127.

8	1	1	2	3	4	2
4	2	6	8	0	8	4
4	2	2	4	1	6	2
5	6	8	0	2	4	4
2	1	4	1	5	0	6
2	4	5	2	7	4	8
4	2	2	2	6	2	4

100. 18, since $18^3 = 5,832$ and $18^4 = 104,976$.

25. Bend over backwards.

163. The middle of nowhere.

84. $\sqrt{(6! + (6! + 6) / 6)} = 29$.

14. 11, 47, and 71.

68. One foot in the grave.

79.

O			X		
			X		
		O			
	X		X		
			O	O	

115. At least two blocks are featured. The first five views are all consistent with each other, but the sixth is not. The "Z" on the upper face would have to be a "U" (with its base at the edge adjoining the face with the "E") for this block to match the others.

32. The traveler on the fast train sees all the trains going the other way around that left up to three hours ago or that will leave in the next two hours. The traveler on the slow train sees all the trains going the other way around that left up to two hours ago or that will leave in the next three hours. In five hours, including the beginning and end, 21 trains depart in each direction. Including the train they are traveling on, each traveler therefore sees 22 trains on his journey.

148. Split level.

36. There are 120 socks in the drawer: 85 red ones and 35 blue ones.

140. Construct the line CG as shown below:

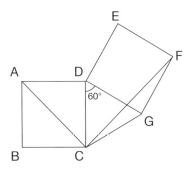

Since DC = DG and angle CDG is 60°, triangle CDG is equilateral, so DC = DG = CG.

Thus, triangle CGF is isosceles, since CG = GF. Angle CGF is angle CGD + angle DGF, which is 60° + 90°, or 150°. So angles GCF and GFC are both 15°.

Since angle DCG is 60° and angle GCF is 15°, angle FCD is 45°. Angle ACD is also 45°, so angle ACF is the sum of FCD and ACD, or 45° + 45°, which is 90°.

80. $6 / (1 - {}^{5}/_{7}) = 21$.

97. The two hands clearly cannot occur in the same deal, so we compare the number of hands that beat these two. They are both beaten by the same number of four-of-a-kinds, but the first hand is beaten by 32 straight flushes, the second by 31. Hence the full house with the three kings is the stronger hand.

158. Three wise men.

128. Five thousand.

114. Queueing.

49. Bermuda Triangle

61.

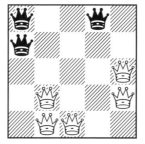

69. The two possible ways of dividing the square are shown below:

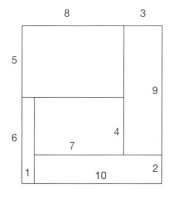 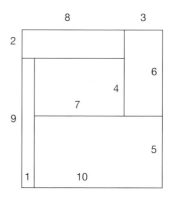

141. They are the same.

Let $S = \sqrt{(12 + \sqrt{(12 + \sqrt{(12 + \sqrt{(12 + \ldots})})})}}$, then $S^2 = 12 + S$, from which $S = 4$. To evaluate

$X = 2 + \sqrt{(2 + \sqrt{(2 + \sqrt{(2 + \sqrt{(2 + \ldots})})})})}$, let

$T = X - 2 = \sqrt{(2 + \sqrt{(2 + \sqrt{(2 + \sqrt{(2 + \ldots})})})})}$.

Then $T^2 = 2 + T$ from which $T = 2$ and $X = 4 = S$.

147. The four ages are 12, 16, 42, and 44.

37. 72 hens, 21 sheep, 7 cows.

89. Unfinished Symphony.

117. $123 - 45 - 67 + 89 = 100$.

48. This puzzle is designed so that most people who see it will think (falsely) that the clues are missing. They think this because they mistake the clues for clue numbers. The clues cannot be the clue numbers, however, since for one thing the puzzle would not then be solvable, and for another the order of the clues has been muddled up.

Clue 21-Across is 21 or, in letters, TWENTY-ONE. Once this clue has been solved the rest are easy. The answer is shown below:

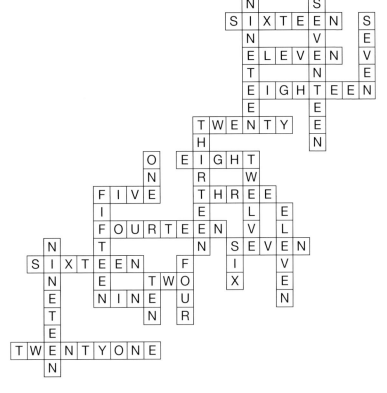

70. 93 and 87. When the digits in each number of the sequence are reversed, the sequence is the multiples of 13; that is, 13, 26, 39, 52, 65, 78, and 91.

119. Let the width of the star be 2a, and construct a line from the center of the star (and circle) to where one of the two outer threads meets the circle.

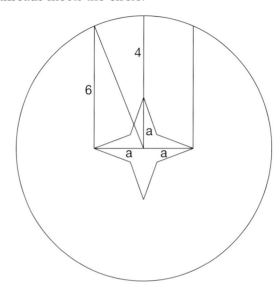

Clearly, the radius of the circle is 4 + a. The diagonal line is a radius, but it is also the hypotenuse of a right-angled triangle with sides of length 6 and a. Thus by the Pythagorean theorem we have $6^2 + a^2 = (4 + a)^2$, so a equals 2.5 cm and the width of the star is 5 cm.

109. The base n of the measurements can be found using the Pythagorean theorem, which gives the following decimal equation: $7^2 + (2n)^2 = (n + 3)^2 + (n + 8)^2$, from which n = 12. Thus the base being used in the question is 12, and using this base, the hypotenuse measures 21. In base 10 the sides are 7, 24, and 25, and 15, 20, and 25.

162. I would not want a tiger to chase me or a zebra to chase me. Given the choice, I'd rather a tiger chased a zebra, not me.

15. TWELVE = 130760, THIRTY = 194215, and NINETY = 848015.

33.

C	D	X	C	I	V	D
L	V	M	M	I	I	L
X	C	I	X	D	X	V
I	C	C	X	C	I	I
C	M	L	X	X	I	X
X	I	I	I	V	C	I
I	X	X	X	I	I	I

64. Noting that the 3-5 domino can be placed uniquely, the full array is soon easily figured out, as shown.

1	2	6	1	6	3	4	5
3	3	6	4	3	2	5	4
3	0	6	0	3	1	2	2
0	5	5	4	6	5	0	2
0	2	5	1	5	0	0	1
6	4	3	4	4	1	1	1
2	2	6	4	5	0	3	6

155. There is no choice regarding the queen and king; each has only one square on which to be placed. The rooks, knights, and bishops can each be positioned in two ways, giving a total of $2^3 = 8$ different combinations. The eight pawns can be positioned in $8! = 40{,}320$ ways. Thus for the pieces of one color there are a total of $8 \times 40{,}320 = 322{,}560$ possibilities.

57. The integers are −3, −1, and 1.

26. The new chart is shown below:

Last week		This week	Last week		This week
Atomic	1	Atomic	Valentine	21	Another Day
Blockbuster	2	Dizzy	What	22	Kayleigh
Classic	3	Footloose	Xanadu	23	Xanadu
Dizzy	4	Blockbuster	YMCA	24	Angie Baby
Emma	5	Jesamine	Zabadak!	25	True
Footloose	6	Classic	Autumn Almanac	26	Mickey
Gaye	7	Night	Angie Baby	27	YMCA
Hello	8	Perfect	Another Day	28	Valentine
Intuition	9	Lamplight	Angel Eyes	29	Angel Eyes
Jesamine	10	Emma	Angel Fingers	30	Ain't Nobody
Kayleigh	11	What	Amateur Hour	31	Amateur Hour
Lamplight	12	Obsession	Angela Jones	32	New entry
Mickey	13	Autumn Almanac	Ain't Nobody	33	Angel Fingers
Night	14	Gaye	American Pie	34	Question
Obsession	15	Reward	Ant Rap	35	Always Yours
Perfect	16	Hello	Alphabet Street	36	Adoration Waltz
Question	17	American Pie	Alternate Title	37	Alternate Title
Reward	18	Intuition	As Usual	38	Sandy
Sandy	19	As Usual	Adoration Waltz	39	Alphabet Street
True	20	Zabadak!	Always Yours	40	Angela Jones

123.

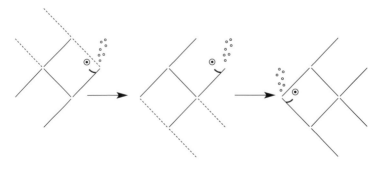

116. See-through blouse.

94.

3	6	1
5	2	9
7	8	4

73. Mate in three can be forced only by **1** d4.

If **1** … Kh5 then **2** Qd3 Kg4 (or Kh4) **3** Qh3 mate.

If **1** … Kg4 then **2** e4+ Kh4 **3** g3 mate.

130.

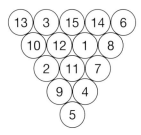

144. Let the longer candle burn at L ^{cm}/_{hr} and the shorter candle at S ^{cm}/_{hr}. Then the longer candle was 8L cm, the shorter candle 8.75S cm, and 8L = 8.75S + 2.

At 8 P.M. the candles were the same length, so 4L = 5S. Solving with the above, S = $^8/_5$ and L = 2, so the longer candle was 16 cm and the shorter candle was 14 cm.

124. Crossroads.

6. Square meal.

76. West Indies.

136. Too few to mention.

74. This is H.E. Dudeney's solution:

1	Nc3	d5
2	Nxd5	Nc6
3	Nxe7	g5
4	Nxc8	Nf6
5	Nxa7	Ne4
6	Nxc6	Nc3
7	Nxd8	Rg8
8	Nxf7	Rg6
9	Nxg5	Re6
10	Nxh7	Nb1
11	Nxf8	Ra3
12	Nxe6	b5
13	Nxc7+	Kf7
14	Nxb5	Kg6
15	Nxa3	Kh5
16	Nxb1	Kh4

22.

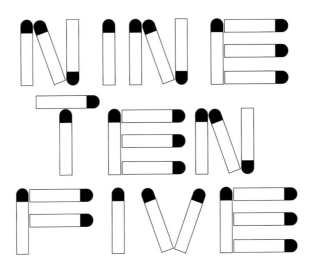

99. Space Invaders.

31. The minimum number of moves made by White's men to reach the position shown in the question is: queen's pawn 5 (d4, c5, b6, a7, a8), new queen 2 (a7, e3), queen's knight 2 (c3, a4), king's knight 2 (f3, h2), king's rook 2 (h3, g3), king's rook's pawn 2 (h3, g4), king's bishop's pawn 1 (f3) and king 1 (f2). These total seventeen and therefore account for all of White's moves. Noting that Black's missing pieces were captured on c5, b6, a7, and g4, the position after White's ninth move would have been as follows:

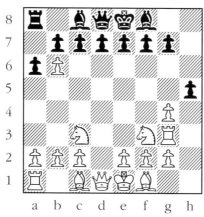

The game from White's ninth move was:

9 ...	Ra7
10 bxa7	h4
11 a8(Q)	h3
12 Qa7	h2
13 Qe3	h1(B)
14 Nh2	a5
15 f3	a4
16 Kf2	a3
17 Na4	

10. e^{π} is greater than π^{e}. To two decimal places, $e^{\pi} = 23.14$ and $\pi^{e} = 22.46$.

134. The values of A, B, and C are 1111, 2222, and 5555, respectively, and the question is whether $B^C + C^B$ is divisible by seven.

$$B^C + C^B = (B^C + C^B) + (4^C - 4^B) - (4^C - 4^B)$$
$$= (B^C + 4^C) + (C^B - 4^B) - 4^B(64^A - 1^A)$$

Since C is odd, $(B^C + 4^C)$ is divisible by $(B + 4)$, which is divisible by seven. $(C^B - 4^B)$ is divisible by $(C - 4)$, which is divisible by seven. Lastly, $4^B(64^A - 1^A)$ is divisible by $(64 - 1)$, which is divisible by seven. Thus $B^C + C^B$ is divisible by seven.

142. Laid back.

95. digital root $(9^{6130} + 2)^{4875}$

$= $ digital root $(2^{4875} + 9 \times (\text{large number}))$

$= $ digital root $(8^{1625} + 9)$

$= $ digital root $((9 - 1)^{1625} + 9)$

$= $ digital root $((9 \times (\text{large number}) - 1) + 9)$

$= $ digital root $(9 - 1 + 9)$

$= 8$

12. By changing his mind, B reduced his chance of winning the game.

The only way in which EEE can appear before OEE is if the first three throws of the die are EEE. Otherwise the sequence EEE must be preceded by an O. The probability of the first three throws being E is $(1/2)^3$, so if B chooses OEE when A has chosen EEE, then B wins with probability $7/8$. If B chooses OOO in response to A's choice of EEE, then B's chance of winning is $1/2$.

4. Each match will eliminate one player, so starting with 89 players will require 88 matches to decide the winner.

53. Just between you and me.

16. A straight-line route that takes the spider one meter down to the floor, forty meters across the floor, and nine meters up toward the ceiling is fifty meters.

Two quicker straight-line routes, found by drawing straight lines from the spider to the fly on a flattened plan of the warehouse, are shown below. The first of these sees the spider heading up the side wall, crossing the ceiling, and finally approaching the fly from above. The distance of this route is $\sqrt{(14^2 + 46^2)} = 48.08$ meters.

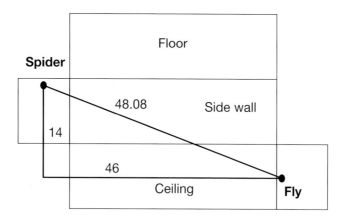

The third straight-line route sees the spider heading diagonally to the floor, then up the side wall, crossing the corner of the ceiling and again at the end approaching the fly from above. The distance of this route is $\sqrt{(20^2 + 42^2)} = 46.52$ meters.

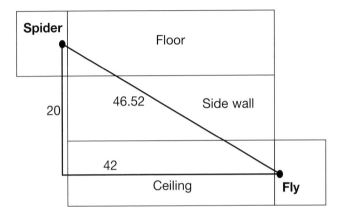

The shortest route is 46.52 meters.

29. The letter m.

50.

$$
\begin{array}{r}
1\ 4\ 5 \\
2\ 0\ 6\ )\ \overline{2\ 9\ 8\ 7\ 0} \\
2\ 0\ 6 \\
\hline
9\ 2\ 7 \\
8\ 2\ 4 \\
\hline
1\ 0\ 3\ 0 \\
1\ 0\ 3\ 0 \\
\hline
\end{array}
$$

258.

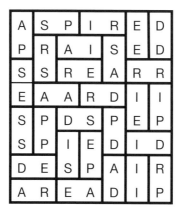

¹A	S	²P	I	R	³E	D
⁴P	R	A	I	⁵S	E	⁶D
⁷S	⁸S	⁹R	¹⁰E	A	R	R
E	A	A	R	D	I	I
S	P	D	S	¹¹P	E	P
¹²S	P	I	E	¹³D	¹⁴I	D
¹⁵D	E	S	P	A	I	R
¹⁶A	R	E	A	¹⁷D	I	P

A	S	P	I	R	E	D
P	R	A	I	S	E	D
S	S	R	E	A	R	R
E	A	A	R	D	I	I
S	P	D	S	P	E	P
S	P	I	E	D	I	D
D	E	S	P	A	I	R
A	R	E	A	D	I	P

Some of the clues explained:

7-Across   The SS were German villains, and the letters SS are found in the center of the word "Russia."

9-Across   To raise a child is to REAR a child; right is R, and someone with musical talent has a good ear.

11-Across	PE (gym class), followed by the first letter of "play," gives you PEP.
12-Across	South Dakota (or SD, for short) is where Pierre is, and if you put pie (dessert) inside, you get SPIED.
14-Across	The id is the unconscious; security guards may ask to see your ID.
16-Across	AREA (region) is contained as a section of the word "Caesarean."
17-Across	"PI'd" reversed give you DIP.
1-Down	If you keep "lapses" (sins) from starting, you get APSES.
2-Down	"Parade is" is an anagram of PARADISE.
3-Down	Erie, Pennsylvania is a homophone of EERIE.
5-Down	"Das" is German for "that"; in hindsight (that is, read backwards), it's SAD.
6-Down	To tear is to rip, D is short for Democrat, and a dullard is a DRIP.
8-Down	To sap is to undermine, so one who undermines is a SAPPER, which is an anagram of "papers."
10-Down	A stanza is a verse; following the introduction of that word is ERSE, which is a Gaelic language.
13-Down	D stands for day, and a spot is an advertisement (or, more briefly, an ad), giving DAD.
14-Down	The initial letters of "Indonesia instigated insurgency" spell III.

232. The area of triangle ABC is $(25\sqrt{3} + 36)$ inches². To show this, consider any two of the triangles making up the equilateral triangle, say ABP and ACP (shown as ACP'). Place the two triangles together, AB on AC, to obtain the figure shown:

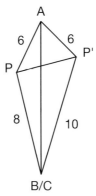

Angles PAB and CAP' total 60°, so PAP' is equilateral. Hence the quadrilateral APBP' can be regarded as an equilateral triangle with 6-inch sides on top of a right-angled triangle with sides 6, 8, and 10 inches. The overall area of the quadrilateral is therefore $(9\sqrt{3} + 24)$ inches².

By taking ABP and BCP, and ACP and BCP, other quadrilaterals can be constructed in a similar manner. Their areas are $(16\sqrt{3} + 24)$ inches² and $(25\sqrt{3} + 24)$ inches² respectively.

The total area of the three quadrilaterals so constructed is $(50\sqrt{3} + 72)$ inches². Because this counts each triangle within the original triangle twice, the area of triangle ABC is therefore $(25\sqrt{3} + 36)$ inches².

280. The missing number is 244,769. This is calculated by adding the number to its left to the product of the two numbers above them; in this case, $6,949 + 1,081 \times 220$. An example from the grid is $220 = 31 + 21 \times 9$.

233. 24 hours in a day
5 vowels in the English alphabet
8 legs on a spider
1,000 words that a picture is worth
13 stripes on the American flag
14 lines in a sonnet
90 degrees in a right angle
9 lives of a cat

229.

	WHITE	BLACK
1.	P–KB3	N–QR3
2.	P–QR4	N–N5
3.	P–Q4	P–QB3
4.	R–R3	Q–R4
5.	R–Q3	N x R mate

The diagram shows the final mate.

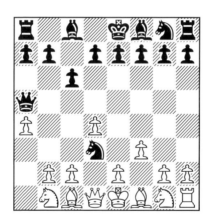

301. The trees are planted as follows:

        X   X

    X   X   X   X

    X   X   X   X

        X   X

235. The number of possible arrangements is 42. To prove this, note that the positions of the 1 and the 9 are fixed. Now suppose that the 2 is placed below the 1. Then if the 3 is placed below the 2, five arrangements are possible. Alternatively, if the 3 is placed to the right of the 1, then there are five arrangements with the 4 under the 2, five with the 5 under the 2, four with the 6 under the 2, and two with the 7 under the 2. This gives a total of 21 arrangements. But by symmetry we would have another 21 if we had started by placing the 2 to the right of the 1, which gives a grand total of 42. (Notice that the digit in the center must be the 4, 5, or 6.)

270. $153 = 1! + 2! + 3! + 4! + 5!$ and $153 = 1^3 + 5^3 + 3^3$. Also, $371 = 3^3 + 7^3 + 1^3$.

171. One solution is shown in the diagram.

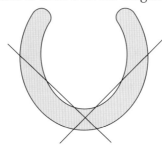

The second solution is to cut the horseshoe into three pieces with one cut, and then put them on top of one another for the next cut. The third solution is to cut the horseshoe in half along the plane of the page, and leaving these pieces on top of one another, cut each of these two pieces into three pieces.

234. Let V $= [\log (1 + \frac{1}{1}) + \log (1 + \frac{1}{2}) + \log (1 + \frac{1}{3})$
$\qquad + ... + \log (1 + \frac{1}{9})] \times 100\%$

Then V $= [\log (\frac{2}{1}) + \log (\frac{3}{2}) + \log (\frac{4}{3}) + ...$
$\qquad + \log (\frac{10}{9})] \times 100\%$
$\qquad = [\log (\frac{2}{1} \times \frac{3}{2} \times \frac{4}{3} \times ... \times \frac{10}{9}] \times 100\%$
$\qquad = [\log (10)] \times 100\%$
$\qquad = 100\%$

207. Luckily for Jimmy, yes!

181. A = buttercup; B = rose (homophone of rows); C = ivy (the clue is in Roman numerals); D = hyacinth (high "a," "c" in "th"). The theme is plants.

173. United States.

178.   29 days in February in a leap year
12 signs of the zodiac
7 wonders of the ancient world
54 cards in a deck (with the jokers)
32 degrees Fahrenheit, at which water freezes
18 holes on a golf course
4 quarts in a gallon
14 pounds in a stone

275. The easiest way to solve this puzzle is to note that the 5 × 5 checkerboard must have 13 squares of one color and 12 of the other. Now, if the cross-shaped piece is excluded, the remaining five pieces comprise 14 white and 11 black squares. Thus the cross-shaped piece must be used.

It is then not too difficult to find the following solution (piece 1 is not used).

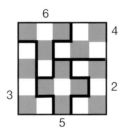

184. Hawaii is the southernmost state and Alaska the northernmost and westernmost state. Less obviously, Alaska is also the easternmost state of the United States. This is because of the Aleutian Islands, which extend from the southwest corner of Alaska's mainland across the line of longitude 180° E/W.

267. Booby prize.

293. Construct a line from O, the center of the pipe, to the foot of the ditch, C, and a radius from O to where the pipe touches one side of the ditch at A. Angle OCA = 60°/2 = 30°, so angle AOC = 60°. Let B be the point where OC crosses the pipe.

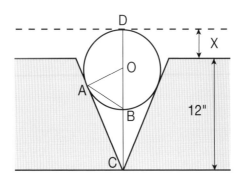

Angle AOB = 60° and OA = OB, so AOB is equilateral and BA = OB = 4.5".

Since angle OAC = 90° and angle OAB = 60°, then angle BAC = 30°.

Thus, BAC is isosceles and BC = BA = OB = 4.5".

DC = DO + OB + BC = 4.5" + 4.5" + 4.5" = (12 + x)".

Thus X, the amount the pipe protrudes above the ground, is 1.5".

269. David, of course. Read the question!

215. Strychnine.

172. A = nose; B = mouth; C = foot; D = spine. The theme is parts of the body.

182. The two lists of words, with the reinserted letters shown uppercase, were as follows: Ado, eBb, CoDE, siFt, Gel, HeIr, JoKe, LuMiNOus, Pig, QuaRtS, TUg, liVe, WaXY, Zest; and doZe, boY, siX, tWelVe, rUT, SoRe, QuiP, ONus, MiLK, JIg, HuG, FatE, gliDe, CaB, eAst.

Minor variations are possible. For example, in the first set of words, "CoDEs, Fit" could replace "CoDE, siFt."

180. 2,025 or 3,025, as $(30 + 25)^2 - (20 + 25)^2 = 3,025 - 2,025 = 1,000$

298. The birthdays being celebrated were 12, 15, and 18. On the first occasion the birthdays being celebrated were 3, 6, and 9. On every birthday the middle child has an age that is half the sum of the other two ages.

205. The position for the cut of the block is shown in the diagram. The side of the cut square is $\sqrt{9^2 + 9^2}$ inches = $\sqrt{(12^2 + 3^2 + 3^2)}$ inches, which is approximately 12.7 inches.

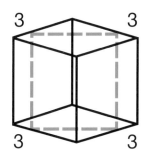

202. Two unrelated women each married the other's son from a previous marriage. Each couple then had a daughter.

268. Britney Spears is an anagram of Presbyterians.

185. One solution is for the digits 0, 1, 2, 3, 4, and 5 to appear on cube one and the digits 0, 1, 2, 6, 7, and 8 to appear on cube two. For dates that include the number 9, simply turn the 6 upside down.

214. Across: 1. Cauldron, 3. Sort, 4. Stifle, 5. Meg Ryan, 6. Envelope, 8. Backwater (O to H is H_2O backwards). Down: 2. Desperation, 7. Edam.

179.

NAME	Mr. Gray	Mr. Brown	Mr. Green	Mr. Black	Mr. White
HOUSE	Blue	Maroon	Mauve	Yellow	Red
TOWN	Wagga Wagga	Woy Woy	Bong Bong	Peka Peka	Aka Aka
TEAM	Waratahs	Brumbies	Sharks	Hurricanes	Crusaders
PET	Kangaroo	Koala	Kookaburra	Kiwi	Kea

Antipodeans may recognize that those who come from Australia have Australian pets and support Australian rugby teams, whereas Mr. White and Mr. Black, the two New Zealanders, have New Zealand pets and support New Zealand rugby teams.

299. A round peg will fill a maximum of $\pi/4 = 78.5\%$ of a square hole. A round hole of unit radius can contain a square peg of maximum side $\sqrt{2}$, and so the square peg will fill a maximum of $2/\pi = 63.7\%$ of a round hole.

Thus, the round peg in a square hole is the better fit.

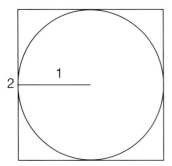
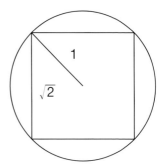

203. A = miner; B = gigolo; C = coroner; D = midwife. The theme is jobs.

191. Each number is put in a column according to the number of letters it has when it is written as a word. The first column contains all the numbers with three letters, the second column has all the numbers with four letters, and so on.

    A. 11 and 12 each have six letters when written as words, and so would appear in the fourth column.

    B. The final entry in the third column would be 60.

186. A = Bronx; B = Broadway; C = Central Park; D = Times Square. The theme is New York City.

197.

N	N	F	X	I	S
E	E	I	O	W	T
I	V	V	N	U	H
G	E	E	E	E	R
H	S	Z	T	L	E
T	W	E	L	V	E

187. True. A tube designed to hold four tennis balls will be half full with two tennis balls and still half full with three tennis balls. This is because the volume of three tennis balls of unit radius is $3 \times \frac{4}{3}\pi = 4\pi$ cubic units, which is half the volume of a cylinder of unit radius and eight units (four tennis balls) high.

289. Labeling the engines, wagons, and different parts of the track as shown will make the solution given here (there is at least one other) easier to follow:

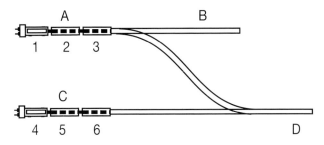

Move 123 to B and uncouple 3. Return 12 to A.

Move 456 to D and uncouple 5 and 6.

Move 12 toward D and couple with 5. Return 125 to A.

Move 125 to B, uncouple 5 and return 12 to A.

Move 12 toward D, leaving 2 in D, where it is picked up by 4 and taken to C.

1 picks up 5 and 3 from B and leaves 3 in D.

42 picks up 3 and returns to C.

Finally 15 picks up 6 from D and returns to A.

276. (a) $1,357 \times 2,468 = 3,349,076$
(b) $8,531 \times 7,642 = 65,193,902$

194. Yes, one, nine, three, nine, three, and nine.

189. Across: 1. Postponed, 3. Other, 4. Astronomer, 5. *HMS Pinafore*, 6. Endearments, 7. A shoplifter, 8. The eyes. Down: 2. The countryside.

288. Apart from its mirror image, the 4×6 solution below is unique.

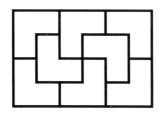

231. D scored no goals against A, and at most one goal against B.

D scored two goals in total, but did not win a game, so D's score against C was 1-1.

D drew against C and so lost to B, so D's score against B was 1-2.

All of B's goals, for and against, were in its match against D, so B's games with A and C were both 0-0.

By subtraction, A's scores against both C and D were 2-0. The results are summarized below:

A vs. B	0-0
A vs. C	2-0
A vs. D	2-0
B vs. C	0-0
B vs. D	2-1
C vs. D	1-1

193. One, one, nine, three, and nine.

196. A = pony; B = dingo; C = sheep; D = lioness. The theme is animals.

239. The fourth clue type is homophones.

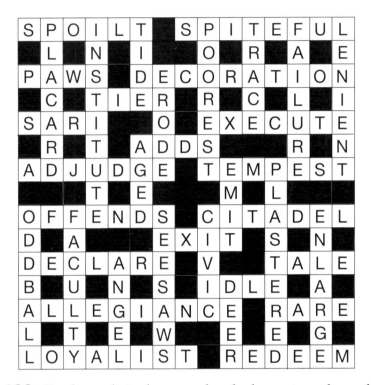

199. Yes, but only in the sense that the letters in each word are in alphabetical order.

188. The numbers correspond to the alphabetical positions of the letters I, V, X, L, D, and M; that is, the letters which are used in Roman numerals written in ascending order of value. The missing letter is "C", which in this sequence corresponds to 3.

198. Mozambique.

168. One set of solutions is:

1. Decade   2. Emblem   3. Sheepish   4. Headache
5. Church   6. Legible   7. Periscope   8. Keepsake

200. It is not possible to end up with just one peg on the board if the central hole starts off empty. To show this, label the holes as shown:

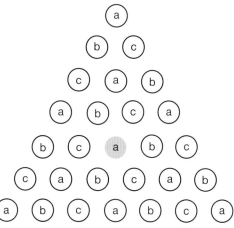

Initially there are nine pegs of each letter. After any move, the number of pegs in two of a, b, and c will be reduced by one, and the number of pegs in the holes of the remaining letter will be increased by one. Thus, at any stage, the amount of pegs assigned to each letter will be either all odd or all even. Hence it is impossible to be left with only one peg on the board, for this would require an odd number (namely one) of pegs in holes of one particular letter and an even number (namely zero) of pegs in the holes of the two other letters.

223. The favorite puzzle books were:

Alan   *Probability Paradoxes*   Emma   *Logic Puzzles*
Ben   *Brain Bafflers*   Fiona   *Mazes*
Claire   *Crosswords*   Gail   *Cryptograms*
Dave   *Number Games*   Henry   *Word Search*

177. A = *Top Gun*; B = *Terms of Endearment*; C = *Born on the Fourth of July* (the "y" is the fourth letter of "July"); D = *Men in Black*. The theme is films.

201. The seven solutions are: 0/0, 1/1, 8/512, 17/4,913, 18/5,832, 26/17,576, and 27/19,683. The four solutions where XSUM is a cube are: 0, 1, 8, and 27.

Note that XSUM = 64 = 4^3 cannot be a solution as X would then need to be at least an eight-digit number, yet 64^3 is only a six-digit number.

208.

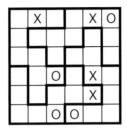

286. Ring D goes over B, which goes over A, which goes over D. Thus, the rubber ring must be A, B, or D. Similarly, B goes over C, which goes over E, which goes over B. The common ring in each case is B, so it must be the rubber one.

167. A = Adam; B = Joseph; C = Richard; D = Justin. The theme is boys' names.

210.

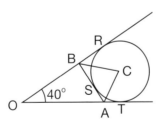

Angle O = 40°, so angles OAB + OBA = 180° – 40° = 140°
Angle TAS = 180° – angle OAB
Angle RBS = 180° – angle OBA
So angles TAS + RBS = 360° – 140° = 220°.
Since CA and CB bisect angles TAS and RBS, respectively,
    angles CAS + CBS = 110°.
Thus, angle ACB = 180° – 110° = 70°.
This angle is independent of the position of the tangent ASB.

169. The semicircle and the tetrahedron are the next two shapes in the series.

The six shapes are a cube, prism, circle, hexagon, cylinder, and rectangle. The number of letters in the name increases by one each time, from four to nine. Of the four shapes from which the seventh and eighth can be chosen, namely a square, tetrahedron, semicircle, and pyramid, only the semicircle and tetrahedron have 10 and 11 letters, respectively.

195.

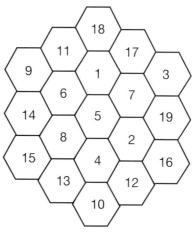

220. Let the dimensions of the hole be x by y inches, then: $1.25(2x + 2y) = xy$, from which $xy - 2.5x - 2.5y = 0$. This may be expressed as $(x - 2.5)(y - 2.5) = 6.25$.

The only integral solutions to this equation are $x = y = 5$, and $x = 15$ and $y = 3$ (or vice versa). Because the hole is wider than it is high, we require the latter solution, so the width of the hole for the letters is 15 inches.

170. Prime numbers of more than one digit end with 1, 3, 7, or 9, as do numbers that are three times prime numbers of more than one digit. Neither the third nor sixth digit of the required ten-digit number can be 7, and 9 cannot appear anywhere in the number. Knowing these facts helps narrow down the possibilities. The required number is 2,412,134,003.

221. 60,481,729, which is $(6,048 + 1,729)^2 = 7,777^2$

212. $73 = \left(\sqrt{\sqrt{\sqrt{4}}} \right)^{4!} + \left(4 \div \overline{.4} \right)$ and $89 = \left(4! \div \sqrt{\overline{.4}} - .4 \right) \div .4$

A line over a decimal indicates that it is a repeating decimal.

245. A. The tire wear after 1,000 miles will be: $1/18 + 1/18 + 1/22 + 1/22 = 20/99$ of a tire. Five tires will therefore last $99/20 \times 5 \times 1,000$ miles = 24,750 miles.

B. Four changes are needed, as shown below:

Miles	Front left	Front right	Rear left	Rear right	Spare
0–6,750	A	B	C	D	E
6,750–11,000	A	E	C	D	B
11,000–13,750	A	E	C	B	D
13,750–18,000	A	E	D	B	C
18,000–24,750	C	E	D	B	A

253. Starting with the lower right empty circle and reading counterclockwise, enter the letters "i," "s," and "t" so that "strategist" can be spelled out.

213. Suppose the army has advanced x miles before the commanding general receives the dispatch. The dispatch rider will then have ridden x + 4 miles.

The dispatch rider now rides $(x + 4) - 4 = x$ miles back to where the army commenced its advance. The rider will arrive at this point at the same time as the rear of the army does and when the front of the army completes its 4-mile advance. Thus, the rider travels 2x + 4 miles while the army travels 4 miles.

Assuming constant speeds throughout, the ratio of the dispatch rider's speed to the army's speed will also be constant. Thus:

$$\frac{x + 4}{x} = \frac{2x + 4}{4}$$

from which $4x + 16 = 2x^2 + 4x$ and $x = \sqrt{8}$

The dispatch rider travels 4 + 2x miles = 9.66 miles.

266. One solution is to weigh $1 + 2 + 3$ against $4 + 5 + 6$, $1 + 5 + 7$ against $2 + 4 + 8$, $1 + 4$ against $2 + 5$, and $3 + 6$ against $7 + 8$. From the results of these four weighings, it can be ascertained which, if any, are the lighter and heavier mince pies.

222. If Jill had said that the number was neither a perfect square nor a perfect cube, then Jack would not have had enough information for an answer. Therefore, Jill must have said that the number was a square or a cube or both. The table below shows the possibilities:

Range	Squares	Cubes	Both
13–499	16, 25, 36, 49, 64, 81,	27, 64	64
	100, 121, 144, 169, 196,	125	
	225, 256, 289, 324, 361,	216	
	400, 441, 484	343	
500–1,300	529, 576, 625, 676, 729,	512	729
	784, 841, 900, 961, 1,024,	729	
	1,089, 1,156, 1,225, 1,296	1,000	

Jill could not have said that the number was a perfect square and a perfect cube; otherwise, Jack could have guessed the number after three questions.

If Jill had said that the number was a perfect square but not a perfect cube, then the fourth question would not have been sufficient to identify the number.

If Jill had said that the number was a perfect cube but not a perfect square, then the fourth question would have been sufficient to identify the number (512 or 1,000) only if Jill had said that the number was not below 500.

Jill therefore answered that the number was not below 500, was not a perfect square, but was a perfect cube. This tells us that the number is below 500, is a perfect square, and is a perfect cube. Therefore, Jill's number is 64.

264. The Statue of Liberty.

224. A = scrambled eggs; B = banana split; C = cutlet; D = antipasto. The theme is food.

285. Remarkably, five queens are still sufficient.

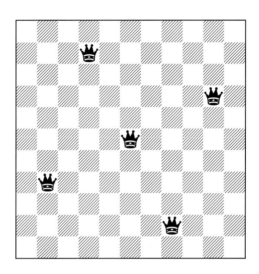

209. A = clarinet; B = pianoforte; C = zither; D = double bass. The theme is musical instruments.

175.

226. Time flies? You cannot–they go too quickly. (If the meaning is still not apparent, "time" is used as a verb and "flies" as a noun.)

176. Across: 2. Parishioners, 3. Point, 4. Past due, 5. An aisle, 6. The Morse code, 7. Twelve + One, 8. Arguments. Down: 1. The nudist colony.

190. A = *The Fifth Element*; B = *What Lies Beneath*; C = *Ghostbusters*; D = *Braveheart*. The theme is films.

216. A = Monica; B = Andrea; C = Stephanie; D = Ingrid. The theme is girls' names.

287. The last-numbered page in the book is number 141, and the missing leaf contains pages 5 and 6. Note that the seemingly alternative solution of the last-numbered page being 142 and the missing leaf being pages 76 and 77 does not work. This is because page 76 would be on the left and page 77 on the right, and therefore on different leaves.

228.

	WHITE	BLACK
1.	P–KB3	N–KB3
2.	P–K4	N x P
3.	Q–K2	N–N6
4.	Q x P ch	Q x Q ch
5.	K–B2	N x R mate

The diagram shows the mate.

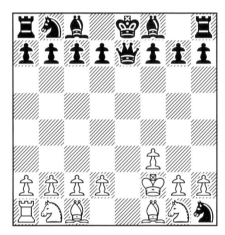

219. N, being the last letter in the word "seven." The sequence is the last letters of the words one, two, three, etc.

217. Alan is from New Ze**alan**d, Rita is from B**rita**in, Eric is from Am**eric**a, and Don is from In**don**esia.

300. $367 \times 52 = 19{,}084$.

291. Starting with the lowest of the three empty circles and reading clockwise, enter the letters "e," "n," and "t" so that "entitlement" can be spelled out.

297. The top left square of the 5×5 grid is 19, and the top left square of the 3×3 grid is 24.

10	49	48	47	8	9	4
11	**19**	37	36	18	15	39
12	20	**24**	29	22	30	38
7	17	23	**25**	27	33	43
44	34	28	21	**26**	16	6
45	35	13	14	32	**31**	5
46	1	2	3	42	41	**40**

240. Apart from using the information given directly, clues can be combined for extra information. For example, clues 1 and 3 can be combined to deduce that Angela is not from Staten Island. Working through, the result below then follows.

MANAGER	ACCOUNT	DISTRICT	CHILDREN
Angela	Aviation	Bronx	4
Brian	Marine	Staten Island	3
Chloe	Liability	New Jersey	5
Dick	Fire	Queens	1
Enid	Automotive	Brooklyn	0
Fred	Property	Manhattan	2

230.

4	2	9	4	1	2	0	9	9	2
7	5	2	9	5	6	4	7	7	4
8	8	1	9	1	1	1	0	5	1
3	1	4	0	3	9	0	2	9	4
1	2	6	2	9	1	9	3	8	4
3	3	0	3	9	2	1	6	4	4

227. The answers to the clues are shown below. In each case, the first word is the one that is to be entered into the diagram:

	M		S		S			D		S		L
P	A	L	E	S	T		S	E	C	U	R	E
	N		D		A			T		I		A
B	I	Z	A	R	R	E		A	L	T	E	R
	L		T		N		I		C		N	
C	A	T	E	R		R	E	L	I	A	N	T
	E				A				S			
D	I	E	T	I	N	G		S	P	E	A	K
I		N		M		E		O		B		
S	C	A	L	P		D	E	P	O	S	I	T
U		G		A		D		D		D		
S	H	E	A	R	S		A	S	L	E	E	P
E		R		T			M		E		S	

ACROSS

7 palest/petals
8 secure/rescue
9 bizarre/brazier
11 alter/later
12 cater/trace
14 reliant/latrine
15 dieting/ignited
17 speak/peaks
20 scalp/claps
21 deposit/topside
23 shears/rashes
24 asleep/elapse

DOWN

1 manila/animal
2 sedate/seated
3 star/arts
4 detail/dilate
5 suitcase/sauciest
6 learnt/rental
10 enraged/angered
13 teenager/generate
15 disuse/issued
16 impart/armpit
18 poodle/looped
19 abides/biased
22 edam/mead

225. The first school had 495 pupils, of whom 286 were boys; the two schools combined had 1,495 pupils, of whom 415 were boys.

237. The first drop should be from floor 14, and the maximum number of drops can be limited to no more than 14.

Suppose the first drop is from floor n. If the crystal breaks, then there is no alternative to dropping the second crystal from floor 1, then floor 2, and so on, up to floor (n – 1) at most. This would ensure that no more than n drops would be required.

Now suppose the crystal does not break on its drop from floor n. The second drop is then from floor (2n – 1), and if the crystal breaks here we start dropping the second crystal from floor n + 1, up to floor (2n – 2) at most. Again this ensures no more than n drops in total.

If the first crystal does not break, we continue advancing up the building by one less floor each time; i.e., by (n – 2), then (n – 3), and so on till we get to the top. We therefore need to find the smallest value of n such that n + (n –1) + (n – 2) + ... + 1 ≥ 105. (Remember, we already know that a crystal dropped from the 106th floor will shatter.)

The sum on the left-hand side simply gives the triangular number $T_n = n(n + 1)/2$, and if $T_n \geq 105$, we then have n(n + 1) ≥ 210. The smallest value of n to satisfy this equation is 14.

273. D = 100. Each letter equals the number in whose name it first appears. Thus tWo, foUr, fiVe, and so on. D first occurs in one hunDreD.

241. Let the train be t minutes early. The wife (driving at 36 mph) saved 5 minutes each way, so the man walked for t – 5 minutes. Because this saved 5 minutes' driving, he walked at 5/(t – 5) of her speed. If she had driven at 46 mph, she would have saved 4 minutes each way, so similar reasoning leads to the equation:

$$\frac{5}{t - 5} \times 36 = \frac{4}{t - 4} \times 46$$

whence t = 50 minutes.

252. A = Orlando; B = Cincinnati; C = New Orleans; D = Washington DC. The theme is American cities.

242.

Aa 7	0	Bb 3	c 1	5
C 8	d 2	1	D 9	e 9
E 4	5	Ff 8	6	4
G 3	2	0	H 7	6

218. THIS = 5,693, THAT = 5,625, IT is 95, and THIS ×
THAT × IT = 3,042,196,875.

238. $119 = \Sigma\Sigma\Sigma\Sigma\sqrt{4} \,/\, \Sigma\Sigma\Sigma\Sigma\sqrt{4} + \Sigma\sqrt{4} = 26{,}796 \,/\, 231 + 3$
$268 = \Sigma(4!) - \sqrt{\sqrt{4}}^{\,\Sigma 4} = 300 - 32$
$336 = \Sigma\Sigma\sqrt{4} \times \Sigma\Sigma 4 + \Sigma\Sigma\sqrt{4} = 6 \times 55 + 6$

All integers from 1 to 336 can be made with three fours
and the symbols given.

265.

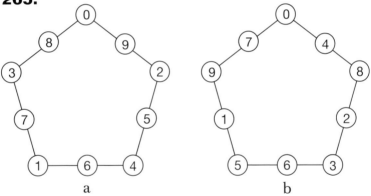

a   b

Other answers to b are possible.

192. The paragraph is unusual because, unlike this answer,
it does not contain the letter "e."

174. Replace each letter in a country's name by the position
of the letter in the alphabet. For example, Italy becomes 9 20
1 12 25. Goals scored is then the smallest difference between
any pair of numbers, so Italy scores 12 − 9 = 3 goals.

The result of the final tie was therefore: Poland 1 Portugal 1.

272.

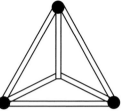

247. Label Samos farm as shown below:

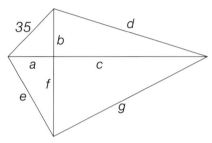

Thus $a^2 + b^2 = 35^2$, $b^2 + c^2 = d^2$, $c^2 + f^2 = g^2$, and $a^2 + f^2 = e^2$, where a, b, c, d, e, f, and g are all different, integral, and not equal to 35.

The unique integral solution to $a^2 + b^2 = 35^2$ is $21^2 + 28^2 = 35^2$. Other integral Pythagorean triangles with a side of 21 or 28 are:

$21^2 + 20^2 = 29^2$ $28^2 + 45^2 = 53^2$

$21^2 + 72^2 = 75^2$ $28^2 + 96^2 = 100^2$

$21^2 + 220^2 = 221^2$ $28^2 + 195^2 = 197^2$

Assuming a is 21 and b is 28 (it does not matter which way around), f is 20, 72, or 220, and c is 45, 96, or 195. Knowing that $\sqrt{(f^2 + c^2)}$ is integral, the only possible values of f and c are 72 and 96. The area of the farm can now be calculated and is: ½ $(21 \times 28 + 21 \times 72 + 96 \times 28 + 96 \times 72)$ / $10 = (21 + 96) \times (28 + 72) / 20 = 585$ acres.

246. The way for Lynsey to win is to play the dashed line shown below. Any other move would allow Heather the opportunity to win.

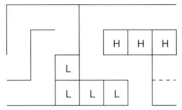

After claiming the two boxes in the bottom right-hand corner, Heather's best move is to open up the nine boxes at the top right and center and hope that Lynsey will take them. Lynsey would be wrong to do so, however, for she can win by the strategy shown below of taking just seven boxes:

Lynsey's sacrifice of two boxes forces Heather to open up the group of ten boxes on the left-hand side for Lynsey. The final result would be as shown below, with Lynsey winning by 21 boxes to 7.

Note that if Lynsey had originally offered Heather the chance of completing the two boxes in the bottom right-hand corner with a vertical line instead of the one shown, Heather could have taken control of the game simply by adding another vertical line to the bottom right-hand corner.

250. 95,759

255.

1	2	7	3	3	6	3	2
1	0	2	4	3	5	6	8
7	2	4	8	8	3	2	0
6	5	6	1	1	1	2	7
9	8	0	1	8	4	6	4
2	1	1	7	6	4	9	8
6	9	6	2	4	1	4	1
1	1	3	8	9	8	9	6

296. A = Connecticut; B = Illinois; C = Wyoming; D = Wisconsin. The theme is U.S. states

251.

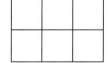

The diagram shows the *ends* of the matches. These are six squares of unit size, and two squares measuring 2 × 2.

249. $3,015,986,724 = 54,918^2$ and $6,714,983,025 = 81,945^2$.

260. Ask A, "Does B tell the truth more often than C?" If the answer is yes, then ask C the next two questions and if the answer is no, ask B. This question is designed to ensure that the second and third questions will not be directed at the man who lies at random.

Question two is: "Do the other two always give the same answer?" As the truthful answer is always "No", this question determines whether the man being asked is the one that is always truthful or the one that always lies.

Question three is: "Of the other two, does A tell the truth more often?" The answer will enable you to determine the status of the other two men.

244. Q is 67,980, and $54{,}321 \times 67{,}980 = 3{,}692{,}741{,}580$.

236.

3	71	5	23
53	11	37	1
17	13	41	31
29	7	19	47

292. $0.56, $1.20, $1.25, $1.50, $1.70, $2.00, and $2.50.

254. White wins as follows:

	WHITE	BLACK
1.	R – QR3	P – N6
2.	R – R1	P x R (Q ch)
3.	Q x Q mate	

257.

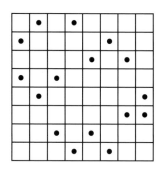

274. The statements can be rewritten as follows:
- Today is Thursday.
- Today is Tuesday.
- Today is Sunday.
- Today is Sunday, Monday, Tuesday, Wednesday, Thursday, or Friday.
- Today is Tuesday.
- Today is Wednesday, Thursday, Friday, or Saturday.
- Today is Monday.

The only day that is not mentioned more than once is Saturday, so today must be Saturday.

259.

¹3	²5	³8	⁴8	⁵9	⁶6
⁷5	3	7	6	0	1
⁸1	2	3	4	6	7
⁹7	9	6	1	5	3
9	7	¹⁰1	7	3	9

10-Across comprises the last four cells of 3-Down, 4-Down, 5-Down, and 6-Down. Each of these is the product of two three-digit primes and therefore ends with 1, 3, 7, or 9. In no answer is a digit repeated, so 10-Across is a four-digit number that is the product of two two-digit primes and contains each of the digits 1, 3, 7, and 9. The only answer for 10-Across that meets these criteria is $37 \times 47 = 1{,}739$. By similar reasoning, 6-Down = 61,739.

The digits of 8-Across are in ascending order, have no digit repeated, and the sixth digit is 7. Using this information and the answers to 6-Down and 10-Across, a computer search will uncover the unique solution.

279. From the information given in the question, we know that the radius of the outer circle (the one on which A and B lie) is three times the radius of the inner, concentric circle through C and D. Thus, the circumference of the outer circle is three times the circumference of the inner circle, and so the arcs AB and CD are equal in length.

Since arc CD is more curved than arc AB, its ends will be closer together. Thus, the lines AC and BD are not parallel–they will meet down and to the left of the diagram.

243. A = goldfinch; B = eagle; C = partridge; D = nightingale. The theme is birds.

281. Vivienne Westwood had 153 outfits exhibited. The "3" represents the number of letters appearing only once in her name (i.e., the "s," "t," and "d"); the "5" represents the number of letters appearing twice (the "v," "i," "n," "w," and "o"); and the "1" represents the number of letters appearing three times (the "e").

284. Suppose n clients were picked, with 10n names in the complete mailing list. The clients picked were numbers 1, 3, 6, 10, ... with the final one being number $n(n + 1)/2$. Since the final one was the last name in the index, it follows that $10n = n(n + 1)/2$, whence $20 = n + 1$. Thus, 19 clients were chosen out of a total mailing list of 190 clients.

261. Begin by noting that the cake's area cannot be less than $(1 \times 10) + (2 \times 9) + (3 \times 8) + (4 \times 7) + (5 \times 6) = 110$ inches². By trial and error, the smallest cake that will meet the requirements will then be found to be 9×13 inches, which has an area of 117 inches². The cut cake is as shown:

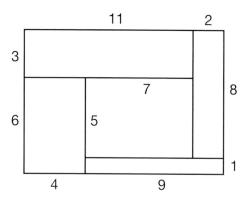

278. Barbara Easton weighs 117 pounds, after losing three pounds.
Anne Frost weighs 113 pounds, after losing two pounds.
Debbie Green weighs 101 pounds, after losing four pounds.
Carol Hope weighs 111 pounds, after gaining one pound.

290. $2 \times \$27 + 2 \times \$34 + \$84 + \$91 = \$297 = 2 \times \$72 + 2 \times \$43 + \$48 + \$19$. The answer is $\$27 + \$34 = \$61$.

282. One solution is:

	3	5	
7	1	8	2
	4	6	

248. As with many puzzles such as this, the flaw is in the given diagram. A more accurate diagram is shown here:

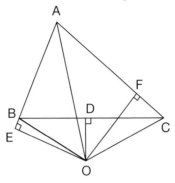

Proceeding as before:

AFO is congruent to AEO, so AE = AF and OE = OF.

BDO is congruent to CDO, so OB = OC.

OEB is congruent to OFC, so EB = FC.

Thus, AE + EB = AF + FC = AC ≠ AB, because AB = AE − EB.

271. A = Hyundai; B = BMW; C = Honda; D = Bentley. The theme is cars.

183. In addition to the information given directly in the question, note that if there is someone who last dined in restaurant A who will be dining next in restaurant B, then the person who last dined in restaurant B cannot be dining next in restaurant A. Working through the information given, the result below then follows:

NAME	CITY	LAST DINNER	NEXT DINNER
Ann	Auckland	Wholemeal Cafe	Farewell Spit Cafe
Ben	Dunedin	Collingwood Tavern	The Old School Cafe
Cathy	Christchurch	Milliways Restaurant	Wholemeal Cafe
David	Wellington	The Old School Cafe	Milliways Restaurant
Emma	Hamilton	Farewell Spit Cafe	Collingwood Tavern

283. The common total is 21. A = 3, B = 4, and C = 5.

262. A = mandolin; B = oboe; C = triangle; D = cymbals (symbols). The theme is musical instruments.

294. The sound of each letter in the top row is the same as a three-letter word that does not include the letter itself: sea, eye, eau (as in eau de Cologne), cue, and ewe.

206.
1. Egypt
2. Qatar
3. Brazil
4. Rwanda
5. Vietnam
6. Senegal
7. Algeria
8. Estonia

256.

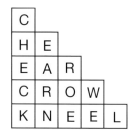

277. The middle circle reads New Zealand, and the five six-letter words are "snooze," "secede," "casino," "meddle," and "Malawi."

295. You might have thought that the camp could have been in the vicinity of the South Pole at any point where a walk one mile east, after the mile south, took the explorer an exact number of times around the South Pole. This would mean that a walk one mile north would then retrace the walk one mile south and the explorer would then be back where she started. However, you would have been wrong, as polar bears do not live at the South Pole!

263. 1! + 4! + 5! = 145.

204. Starting with the empty circle on the right and reading counterclockwise, enter the letters "u," "n," and "d" so that "underground" can be spelled out. The less common word "undergrounder" is also formed from this circle.

211. The equation TIM × SOLE = AMOUNT is sufficient, with a computer search, to solve this puzzle. However, the extra information provided enables the puzzle to be solved as follows:

Because LEAST and MOST both end in ST, and either LEAST – MOST = ALL or MOST – LEAST = ALL, then L = 0.

Substituting L = 0 in LEAST – MOST = ALL and MOST – LEAST = ALL, then either EA – MO = A or MO – EA = A.

As L = 0, then O ≠ 0 so EA – MO ≠ A and MO – EA = A. From this, MO = EA + A, M = E + 1, and O is even. As L = 0, O = 2, 4, 6, or 8 and A = 6, 7, 8, or 9.

As TIM × SOLE = AMOUNT, then M × E is a number that ends with T. As we also know that M = E + 1, then T = 2 or 6. (Note that T ≠ 0 because L = 0.)

If T = 6, then S = 1 since TIM × SOLE is a six-digit number and E = 2 or 7.

If T = 6 and E = 2, then M = 3, S = 1 (see above), and O = 4 or 8. O ≠ 8, since TIM × SOLE is a six-digit number, and if O = 4, A = 7 and there is no solution, so this combination is eliminated.

If T = 6 and E = 7, then M = 8. However, then A = 9 and O = 8, which is impossible because M = 8. This combination is therefore also eliminated, and T = 2 because T ≠ 6.

Given that T = 2, then E = 3, 6, or 8 with corresponding values for M of 4, 7, and 9. Also, as T = 2, then O ≠ 2, so O = 4, 6, or 8 and A = 7, 8, or 9.

If E = 3 and M = 4, then S = 1 as TIM × SOLE is a six-digit number. But T = 2 and S = 1 implies A is less than 6, and A = 7, 8, or 9, so this combination is eliminated.

If E = 8 and M = 9, then A = 7 and O = 4. As TIM × SOLE is a six-digit number, S = 1 or 3, but then there is no solution, so this combination is eliminated.

Therefore L = 0, T = 2, E = 6, M = 7, O = 8, A = 9, and S = 3, from which I = 5, U = 1, and N = 4, giving 257 × 3,806 = 978,142.

417. Label the triangle as shown and let the area of △ADO be P acres and that of △AOE be Q acres:

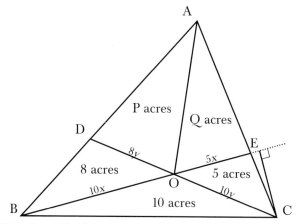

The formula for the area of a triangle is half the base times the perpendicular height. The perpendicular height to C for triangles △OEC and △BEC are the same (both are represented by the line reaching from point C to the extension of line BE), so the lengths of those triangles' bases will be in direct proportion to their areas. Thus if OE is $5x$, then BE is $15x$ and BO is $10x$. Similarly, if DO is $8y$, then DC is $18y$ and OC is $10y$. Using the same technique:

$$\frac{P}{8y} = \frac{Q+5}{10y} \text{ and } \frac{Q}{5x} = \frac{P+8}{10x}$$

Thus $5P = 4Q + 20$ and $2Q = P + 8$, from which $P = 12$ and $Q = 10$. The required answer is $P + Q$, which is 22 acres.

403. All the letters in the series are capital letters without curves. The next term is L.

343. The letters represent the arrangement of men on a chessboard (rook, knight, bishop, queen, king, bishop, knight, rook) in standard chess notation, so the type of music that's missing is Rhythm and Blues (R&B).

311. First, visualize the problem this way:

$$1\ 1\ 1\ 1\ 1\ 1\ 1\ 1\ 1\ 1 = 10$$

Between the first two digits, you may or may not place a plus sign. The same choice applies to the second and third digits, the third and fourth, and so on. As long as you place at least one plus sign, you will have a possible solution. For example, here is a way of placing plus signs that is equivalent to $2 + 3 + 1 + 4$:

$$1\ 1 + 1\ 1\ 1 + 1 + 1\ 1\ 1 = 10$$

There are $2^9 = 512$ ways of placing the plus signs, including the special situation of placing none. Therefore there are $512 - 1 = 511$ equations for the kindergarten to use. As they have wall space for only 500 equations, they cannot show all the solutions.

367.

4	6	3	7	2	6	4
5	5	4	7	2	1	2
1	1	1	7	1	1	1
3	3	5	7	2	3	3
1	4	2	7	2	5	5
6	6	6	7	6	6	6
3	3	3	7	2	5	4
4	4	4	7	2	5	5

382. $111 = 135 - 24$ $666 = (5 \times 4 \div .1 - .2) \div .3$
$222 = 214 + 3 + 5$ $777 = (5 \times 31 + .4) \div .2$
$333 = 345 - 12$ $888 = (15^2 - 3) \times 4$
$444 = (152 - 4) \times 3$ $999 = (5^3 \times 4 \times 2) - 1$
$555 = 542 + 13$

331. Ronald Reagan.

419. Turn two switches on for one minute, then turn one of them off and leave the booth.

- If the green bulb is on, then the switch that is still on is the one that controls the green bulb.
- If the green bulb is off but hot to the touch, then the switch that you just turned off is the one that controls the green bulb.
- If the green bulb is off and cool to the touch, then the switch that controls it is the one that was never turned on.

359.

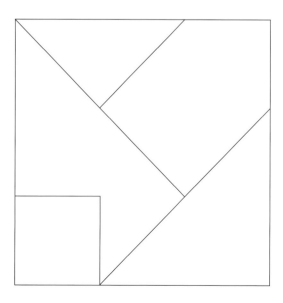

371. The lowest number is 34,217 (equals 102,651 in base eight) and the highest is 250,148 (equals 750,444 in base eight).

400. TED = 682 and VINDICATE = 317,214,568. Thus VIC is 2 × IAN because 314 = 2 × 157.

310. The innkeeper of the "Rose & Crown" is talking to a sign painter and is saying "There is too much space between 'Rose' and '&' and '&' and 'Crown.'"

325. 149, 263, and 587.

376. Only five points are needed, as shown in the example below:

	Your hand	Opponent 1	Dummy	Opponent 2
♣	10 9 8 7 5 4 2	A K Q J	—	6 3
♦	—	J 10 9 8	5 4 3 2	A K Q 7 6
♥	—	A J 3 2	10 9 8 7	K Q 6 5 4
♠	A 10 8 6 4 2	K	J 9 7 5 3	Q

Spades are trump. If the defense leads with a diamond or heart, ruff with a low spade and lead the ace of spades. If the defense leads a trump, win with the ace and lead a club for dummy to ruff. If the defense leads a club, ruff in dummy, then lead a trump to your ace.

Continue leading any suit other than spades and cross-ruffing. After the dummy wins the fourth club lead with a ruff, dummy will have no trumps left. You ruff dummy's lead one last time, and then whatever card you lead cannot be beaten.

409. Lemon meringue.

345. Take 9 coins from bag A, 12 from bag B, and 13 from bag C. No coins are taken from bag D. Weigh these coins and calculate the difference between their weight and the weight of 34 genuine coins. Each possible difference can be accounted for with only one pairing of bags (as explained in the table below), making it possible to identify which bags contain counterfeit coins.

In the table below, "A + 2B" indicates that the coins in bag A were overweight or underweight by one gram, and that the coins in bag B were overweight or underweight (whichever is the same as bag A) by two grams. Similarly, "A – B" means that the coins in bag A were overweight or underweight by one gram, and that the coins in bag B were underweight or overweight (whichever is the *opposite* of bag A) by one gram. When D is one of the counterfeit bags, all we know about it is that the coins in it are counterfeit; we don't know whether they are overweight or underweight.

1	B – C	12	B + D	26	2C + D
2	2B – 2C	13	C + D	30	2A + B
3	A – B	14	B – 2C	31	2A + C
4	A – C	15	A – 2B	33	A + 2B
5	2A – C	17	A – 2C	35	A + 2C
6	2A – B or	18	2A + D	37	2B + C
	2A – 2B	21	A + B	38	B + 2C
8	2A – 2C	22	A + C	42	2A + 2B
9	A + D	24	2B + D	44	2A + 2C
11	2B – C	25	B + C	50	2B + 2C

365. There were eight people at the gathering before Vanessa arrived, for a total of 28 handshakes. Vanessa knew seven of the eight other people at the party.

393.

$$
\begin{array}{r}
1\ 7\ 9 \\
\times\ \ 2\ 2\ 4 \\
\hline
7\ 1\ 6 \\
3\ 5\ 8\ \ \\
3\ 5\ 8\ \ \ \\
\hline
4\ 0\ 0\ 9\ 6
\end{array}
$$

411. The contestant should swap the chosen envelope for the other one.

He will only lose the grand prize if he chose it originally. If he chose the wrong envelope (which he has a two-thirds chance of doing), the host will open the other non-winning envelope, leaving the one holding the grand prize. So swapping envelopes gives the contestant a two-thirds chance of winning the grand prize. If you're not convinced this answer is correct, experiment with envelopes of your own and see what happens!

326. The numbers in the column on the left have an odd number of letters, while the numbers in the column on the right have an even number of letters. As "one million" contains an even number of letters, it belongs in the second group.

384.

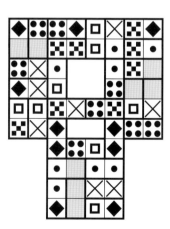

370. Let C be on LB such that ∠CAL = ∠ABL.

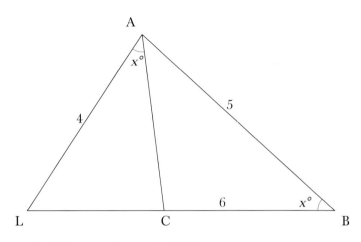

 △CAL is similar to △ABL because:
  ∠CAL = ∠ABL (by construction)
  ∠CLA = ∠BLA (same angle)
  ∠ACL = ∠BAL (180° − $x°$ − ∠L)

 The sides opposite angles ∠ACL and ∠BAL are in the ratio 2 to 3, so each side of △CAL is two-thirds of the length of the corresponding side of △ABL. Thus CA = $^{10}/_3$ and LC = $^8/_3$. So CB = LB − LC = $^{10}/_3$ = CA, which means △BCA is isosceles and ∠BAC = ∠ABC = $x°$. Thus ∠A is $x° + x° = 2x°$ = twice ∠B.

392. The average speed in the first second is 12 inches per second, so assuming constant acceleration, the car's speed at the end of the first second was 24 inches per second. At the end of five seconds, the car would have accelerated to $5 \times 24 = 120$ inches per second for an average speed over the 5 seconds of 60 inches per second. The distance covered in 5 seconds is therefore 300 inches or 25 feet.

315. The numbers on the right are ascending powers of two. The answer to the first equation was given as an example. The rest are: **12** (Angry Men) − **10** (Fingers on a Pair of Gloves) = **2** (Sides to Every Story); **29** (Days in February in a Leap Year) − **25** (Years of Marriage in a Silver Anniversary) = **4** (Suits in a Deck of Cards); **3** (Goals in a Hat Trick) + **5** (Rings on the Olympic Flag) = **8** (Legs on a Spider); **20** (Numbers on a Dartboard) − **4** (Quarts in a Gallon) = **16** (Ounces in a Pound); **18** (Holes on a Golf Course) + **14** (Days in a Fortnight) = **32** (Degrees Fahrenheit at which Water Freezes); **90** (Degrees in a Right Angle) − **26** (Letters of the Alphabet) = **64** (Squares on a Chessboard).

416. Snow blower (S, no W, B lower).

389. Adjacent missiles start the journey $\sqrt{(50^2 + 50^2)} = 70.71$ miles apart, and by symmetry move at a constant 90° angle to their neighbor. Therefore, with a range of only 70 miles, the missiles will not collide and the fighting unit's base will not be destroyed.

328. The two pieces of land are shaped like so:

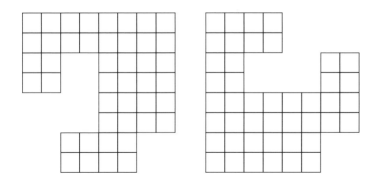

372. Each person consumed eight items, so Tom sold seven items to Harry and Dick sold one. Thus Tom should receive seven coins from Harry and Dick just one.

355. You don't need to know the location of Secret Place to find the treasure. Wherever you stand to follow the instructions, you will end up directly over the treasure. It is buried at a point that can also be found by walking half the distance from Crossbones Rock to Hangman's Tree, turning 90° left, and walking the same distance again.

406. The center of each tree forms a right triangle with the ends of the hedge (as does any point on the curved side). The problem is thus to find an integer less than 1,760 whose square can be expressed as the sum of two nonzero squares in 13 different ways. That integer is 1,105, so the hedge is 1,105 yards long.

Measurements from the first 13 trees to the hedge are (47, 1,104); (105, 1,100); (169, 1,092); (264, 1,073); (272, 1,071); (425, 1,020); (468, 1,001); (520, 975); (561, 952); (576, 943); (663, 884); (700, 855); and (744, 817). The measurements for the other 13 trees are the same, but with the order of the measurements reversed.

302.

$$\left(\sqrt{\frac{1}{.1}} + 1\right)! = 24 \qquad 22 + 2 = 24 \qquad 3^3 - 3 = 24$$

$$\left(4 + \sqrt{4}\right) \times 4 = 24 \qquad 5! \div \left(\sqrt{5} \times \sqrt{5}\right) = 24$$

$$6 \times 6 \times .\overline{6} = 24 \qquad \left(7 - \sqrt{\frac{7}{.7}}\right)! = 24$$

$$8 + 8 + 8 = 24 \qquad 9 \times \sqrt{9} - \sqrt{9} = 24$$

Some alternate solutions are possible.

312. Two solutions, each using four pourings, are:

	11-cup jug	13-cup jug	17-cup jug
Contents at start	9	9	9
After 1 pour	5	13	9
After 2 pours	0	13	14
After 3 pours	11	2	14
After 4 pours	8	2	17

	11-cup jug	13-cup jug	17-cup jug
Contents at start	9	9	9
After 1 pour	1	9	17
After 2 pours	0	10	17
After 3 pours	11	10	6
After 4 pours	8	13	6

322. $10^5 = 10 \times 10^4 = (1 + 9) \times 10^4 = (1^2 + 3^2) \times 100^2 = 100^2 + 300^2$. There are two other pairs of squares that add up to 100,000 ($12^2 + 316^2$ and $180^2 + 260^2$), but they're not easily found without a computer.

For the second question, we are told that 17 is the only prime factor of 1,419,857. After factoring, we find that $1,419,857 = 17^5$. Proceeding as before, $1,419,857 = (1 + 16) \times 17^4 = (1^2 + 4^2) \times 289^2 = 289^2 + 1,156^2$. (Other, harder-to-find solutions are $404^2 + 1,121^2$ and $799^2 + 884^2$.)

386. The series can be rewritten as $1^2 + 1^3$, $2^2 + 2^3$, $3^2 + 3^3$, $4^2 + 4^3$, $5^2 + 5^3$, and so on. The next term is therefore $6^2 + 6^3$, which equals 252.

338. *Stuart Little.*

329. From the diagram given, construct point A such that AD = CD and ∠ADC is 90°, and extend BD to point E such that DE = BD.

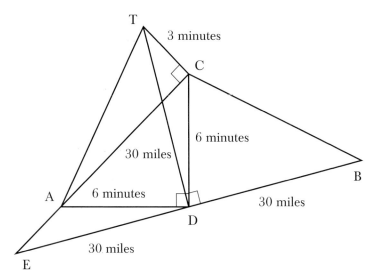

T

3 minutes

C

6 minutes

30 miles

B

A

6 minutes

30 miles

D

30 miles

E

△CDA is isosceles and ∠CDA is a right angle, so ∠ACD is 45° and ∠ACT = 135° − 45° = 90°.

AC = $\sqrt{(6^2 + 6^2)}$ = $\sqrt{72}$ minutes of flying time. TA = $\sqrt{(3^2 + 72)}$ = 9 minutes of flying time.

∠EDA = ∠TDC (since both are equal to ∠EDC − 90°), so △EDA and △TDC are congruent. By symmetry, BC = TA, and flying the distance BC will take 9 minutes.

379. The letters in NEW DOOR can be rearranged to spell the phrase "ONE WORD."

356. 134,689 = 367².

394. The two solutions are 1,787,109,376 and 8,212,890,625.

346. Since the first player could not determine the color of the ball in box 2, boxes 1 and 3 must have contained red/yellow, yellow/red, or red/red. (If they had contained yellow/yellow, he would have known box 2 contained a red ball.)

If box 3 had contained a yellow ball, the second player would have been able to determine that box 1 contained a red ball. Since he could not do so, box 3 must contain a red ball.

308. The complete division is:

$$
\begin{array}{r}
9\ 0\ 8\ 0\ 9 \\
1\ 2\ \overline{)\ 1\ 0\ 8\ 9\ 7\ 1\ 0} \\
\underline{1\ 0\ 8} \\
9\ 7 \\
\underline{9\ 6} \\
1\ 1\ 0 \\
\underline{1\ 0\ 8} \\
2
\end{array}
$$

410. The monks and nuns received more than $56,000 each. If there were five of them, they would receive only $48,000 each, so there must be one, two, three, or four of them, each receiving $240,000, $120,000, $80,000, or $60,000 respectively. Subtracting $56,000 from those amounts gives $184,000, $64,000, $24,000, and $4,000.

Only $24,000 and $4,000 divide evenly into $240,000, so the number of monks and nuns must be three or four. But the number can't be three, since we're told that the monks received the same amount of money as the nuns, so the number must be even. Therefore, there were 60 grandchildren ($240,000 ÷ $4,000), two of whom were monks and two of whom were nuns.

332. Yes; 77 gives the chain $77 \rightarrow 49 \rightarrow 36 \rightarrow 18 \rightarrow 8$. There is no other two-digit number that requires more than three multiplications.

366. Linda, Marlene, Madeline, Nora. The theme is "women's names."

396. Leaning Tower of Pisa.

323. $138 \times 138 = 19,044.$

349. a)

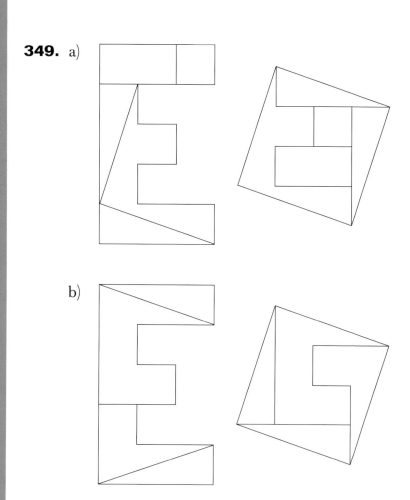

b)

404. If we redraw the circuit as below, the answer is easier to see:

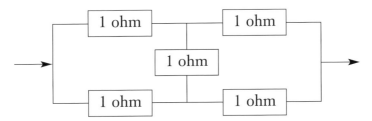

The resistance is $.5 \times 2 = 1$ ohm. The middle resistor has no effect.

387. Raised eyebrows.

340. Label the columns A, B, C, and D from left to right, and the rows 1, 2, 3, and 4 from top to bottom. One solution is as follows:

> Move the tile at A1 to the bottom of the column.
> Move the tile at A2 to the right end of the row.
> Move the tile at A1 to the bottom of the column.
> Move the tile at B4 to the left end of the row.
> Move the tile at C3 to the top of the column.
> Move the tile at A1 to the right end of the row.
> Move the tile at D1 to the bottom of the column.
> Move the tile at B2 to the right end of the row.

309. The numbers in the series, spelled out, are one, two, four, five, seven, eight, eleven, twelve, thirteen, fourteen, fifteen, and sixteen. Taking these numbers in pairs, each has the same number of letters as the other. The next four numbers are therefore eighteen, nineteen, twenty-one, and twenty-two.

374. Abraham Lincoln.

408. If the first cube had been totally submerged before the second cube was placed on the pond floor, then the second cube would also have raised the water level by three inches. The second cube raised the water level by four inches, so the first cube was not totally submerged before the second cube was placed.

If the first two cubes had been totally submerged before the third cube was placed on the pond floor, then the third cube would have raised the water level by less than four inches. This is the case because it would have taken the submersion of all of cube two *and* part of cube one to raise the water level four inches. Therefore the first and second cubes were not fully submerged when the third cube was placed.

If the three cubes were not fully submerged after the third cube was placed, then the water level would have risen by more than four inches. As the water level did not rise by more than four inches, all three cubes must have been submerged once the third cube was placed on the pond floor.

Let A be the area of the pond's base, s be the length of one of the cube's sides, and x be the depth of the pond before the cubes were added. We then have:

$$3A = s^2(x + 3)$$
$$7A = s^2(x + 7) + s^2(x + 7)$$
$$11A = s^3 + s^3 + s^3$$

Multiplying the first equation by 7 and the second equation by 3, and then dividing each by s^2, we get $7x + 21 = 6x + 42$, hence $x = 21$.

Substituting for x in the first equation, A $= 8s^2$, and substituting for A in the third equation, $s = 11 \times 8 \div 3$, or 29.33 inches.

(For the sake of completeness, A $= 8s^2 = 8 \times 29.33^2$ square inches $= 47.8$ square feet.)

353. The fifth man received 2,302 coconuts. From the starting pile of 15,621 coconuts, the first man received 4,147 coconuts, the second man 3,522 coconuts, the third man 3,022 coconuts, and the fourth man 2,622 coconuts. The remaining six coconuts went to the monkey.

333.

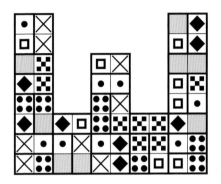

381. $^{5}/_{34} + ^{7}/_{68} + ^{9}/_{12} = 1$

317.

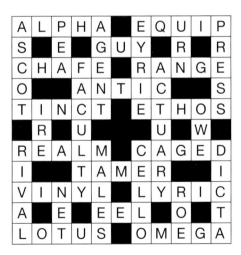

A	L	P	H	A		E	Q	U	I	P
S		E		G	U	Y		R		R
C	H	A	F	E		R	A	N	G	E
O			A	N	T	I	C			S
T	I	N	C	T		E	T	H	O	S
	R		U				U		W	
R	E	A	L	M		C	A	G	E	D
I			T	A	M	E	R			I
V	I	N	Y	L		L	Y	R	I	C
A		E		E	E	L		O		T
L	O	T	U	S		O	M	E	G	A

395. The answer is 111,111,111, and is guessable given this pattern: $11^2 = 121$; $111^2 = 12,321$; $1,111^2 = 1,234,321$; etc.

303. The maximum number of properties owned by Donald is 27 (10 + 9 + 8) and the minimum is 6 (3 + 2 + 1). The number of possibilities for sharing from 6 to 27 properties among three people with no two having the same number of properties is 120.

Since we are told that knowing the total number of properties is insufficient for the daughters to deduce the three inheritances, totals of 6, 7, 26, and 27 can be eliminated immediately. That leaves 116 possibilities.

The eldest daughter is initially unable to deduce the inheritance of her two sisters. This eliminates combinations such as 8/7/5, where the eldest daughter, knowing both the amount of her own inheritance and the total number of properties, could have deduced each of her sister's inheritances. This brings us to 92 possibilities.

Continuing in this vein, after six "no" answers, we have 30 possibilities:

Total	Possible combinations for each total
15	9/5/1, 9/4/2, 8/6/1, 8/5/2, 8/4/3, 7/6/2, 7/5/3
16	10/5/1, 10/4/2, 9/6/1, 9/5/2, 9/4/3, 8/6/2, 8/5/3
17	10/6/1, 10/5/2, 9/7/1, 9/6/2, 9/5/3, 8/7/2, 8/6/3
18	10/6/2, 10/5/3, 9/7/2, 9/6/3, 9/5/4, 8/7/3, 8/6/4
19	10/6/3, 9/7/3

Because the eldest daughter was able to deduce the inheritance of her two sisters at this stage, we can deduce that the total inheritance was 19 properties. To determine whether the distribution was 10/6/3 or 9/7/3, we must look at the eldest daughter's statement that the last two answers (both "no") gave her some information, and see what she would have deduced, knowing that the total inheritance was 19 properties.

	Possibilities remaining
After 4 noes	10/7/2, 10/6/3, 9/8/2, 9/7/3, 9/6/4
After 5 noes	10/7/2, 10/6/3, 9/7/3, 9/6/4
After 6 noes	10/6/3, 9/7/3

Although the fifth "no" helps us (allowing us to eliminate the combination 9/8/2), it would only have provided information to the eldest daughter if she had been told she was inheriting nine properties. Thus the answer is nine properties for the eldest daughter, seven for the middle daughter, and three for the youngest.

363. The numbers used are the first six even numbers. The answer to the first equation was given as an example. The rest are: **4** (Seasons in a Year, Sides on a Square, Faces on Mount Rushmore); **6** (Feet in a Fathom, Pockets on a Pool Table, Characters in Search of an Author); **8** (Arms on an Octopus, King Henrys of England, Pints in a Gallon); **10** (Pins in a Bowling Alley, Years in a Decade, Little Indians); **12** (Inches in a Foot, Signs of the Zodiac, Disciples of Christ or Days of Christmas).

339. H O T
A R E
S E E

402. Although the gravity is lower on the moon than on Earth, a helicopter cannot fly on the moon as it would have no atmosphere to fly in!

347. There is just one, measuring 6 × 8 × 10.

319. $854 = \sqrt{729{,}316}$.

341. Twenty hexagons and twelve pentagons have $20 \times 6 + 12 \times 5 = 180$ sides between them. Each side is paired with another when sewn, giving 90 pairs of edges to be stitched. The length of thread needed is therefore $90 \times 5 = 450$ inches.

383. $5^3 + 3^3 + 3^3 + 3^3 + 2^3 + 2^3 + 2^3 + 2^3 + 1^3 = 239$

$4^3 + 4^3 + 3^3 + 3^3 + 3^3 + 3^3 + 1^3 + 1^3 + 1^3 = 239$

307.

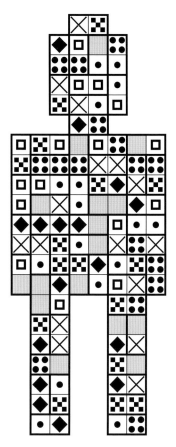

375. $(1 + 2 - 3 - 4) \times (5 - 6 - 7 - 8 - 9) = 100$. (Other solutions are possible.)

330. The sides of the triangle measure 9, 10, and 17 units.

407. The digits of the code are in alphabetical order. The middle digits are 17.

391. 8π inches, or just over two feet.

335. A domino placed on a chessboard will cover one white square and one black square, so 31 dominoes placed on a chessboard must cover 31 squares of each color. The board described has 30 squares of one color and 32 of the other, so the answer is "no."

358. The terms in the series are 10 in base 10, 20 in base 9, 30 in base 8, and so on. The next term in the series is 70 in base 4, which is 1,012.

320.

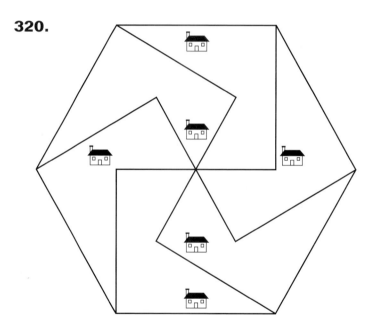

334. Let F be on AD such that CF = CD.

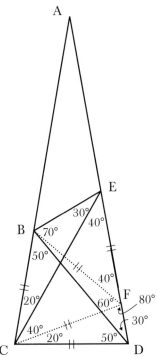

△FCD is isosceles, so ∠CFD = 80°, ∠FCD = 20°, and ∠ECF = 40° (∠ECD's 60° − ∠FCD's 20°).

The angles of a triangle total 180°, so ∠CBD = 50° and ∠CED = 40°. ∠CDB = ∠CBD, so △CBD is isosceles and CD = CB.

Since CF = CD, CF = CB and ∠CBF = ∠CFB = ½(180° − ∠BCF) = 60°. △CBF is therefore equilateral and CB = BF = CF.

∠ECF = ∠CEF, so △ECF is isosceles and CF = EF.

∠EFB = 40° (180° − ∠CFB's 60° − ∠CFD's 80°). Since BF = CF, BF = EF and △BEF is isosceles, so ∠EBF = ∠BEF = ½(180° − ∠EFB) = 70°.

Thus ∠BEC = ∠BEF − ∠CEF = 70° − 40° = 30°.

318. From the information about the alternative routes home from the shopping mall, the shopper must live somewhere on the highlighted section or at the circled point in the first diagram below. The information about the position of the cafe then enables both the site of the cafe and the shopper's home to be determined as shown in the second diagram.

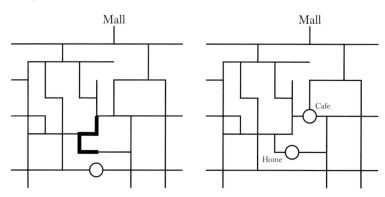

361. The answer is 204 squares. There is one square measuring 8×8, 2^2 squares measuring 7×7, 3^2 squares measuring 6×6, and so on up to 8^2 squares measuring 1×1. This gives a total of $1 + 2^2 + 3^2 + 4^2 + 5^2 + 6^2 + 7^2 + 8^2 = 204$.

414. Here's a lesson in water safety: Susie will not be able to swim back! The current doubled her speed while swimming to the boat, so when swimming against the current, she will make no progress whatsoever.

350. Khaki = arks. The key is to replace each letter with the number that represents its position in the alphabet, and then close up the gaps and respace to make a new word. For example, "beer" is equivalent to "yeah" because beer = 2 5 5 18 = 25518 = 25 5 1 8 = yeah. Hence khaki = 11 8 1 11 9 = 1181119 = 1 18 11 19 = arks.

304. The number 4 is a perfect square.

398. To identify the integers we are told that we would have to know their product and the smallest integer. Since knowledge of the product by itself would not allow us to determine the four integers, the product must be obtainable in more than one way. A list of such integers whose factors total less than 18 is given below.

If the smallest integer were 1, then knowledge of this fact with knowledge of the product would still not be sufficient to determine the four integers. Therefore the smallest integer cannot be 1 and, by elimination, must be 2. It follows that the product is 120 and the integers are 2, 3, 4, and 5.

Product	1st possibility	2nd possibility	3rd possibility
48	1, 2, 3, 8	1, 2, 4, 6	
60	1, 2, 3, 10	1, 2, 5, 6	1, 3, 4, 5
72	1, 2, 4, 9	1, 3, 4, 6	
80	1, 2, 4, 10	1, 2, 5, 8	
84	1, 2, 6, 7	1, 3, 4, 7	
90	1, 2, 5, 9	1, 3, 5, 6	
96	1, 2, 6, 8	1, 3, 4, 8	
120	1, 3, 5, 8	1, 4, 5, 6	2, 3, 4, 5

354. The sum of the fourth powers of the digits in the number equals the number. For example, $1^4 + 6^4 + 3^4 + 4^4 = 1 + 1{,}296 + 81 + 256 = 1{,}634$.

420. The Spice Girls.

336. One solution is to run a fence from C to B, and another fence from A to E (the midpoint of CD). In the diagram below, Y is the intersection of AE and BC, and X and Z are the feet of the perpendiculars from Y to AB and CD respectively.

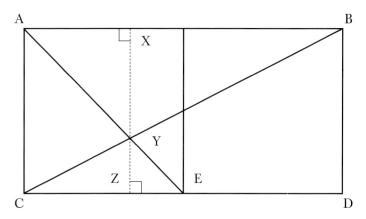

∠CYE = ∠AYB and ∠CEY = ∠BAY, so △CEY and △BAY are similar.

Since AB is twice CE, XY is twice YZ. Therefore YZ = XZ ÷ 3 = AC ÷ 3.

The area of △CEY is ⅓AC × ½CD × ½ = ⅓ × ½ × ½ × (AC × CD) = ⅓ × ½ × ½ × 12 acres = 1 acre.

The area of △ABY is four times that of △CEY (since AB is twice CE and XY is twice YZ) and is therefore 4 acres.

The area of △ACE is one-fourth of ▭ABCD and is therefore 3 acres, so we know that △ACY has an area of 2 acres (since △ACY + △CEY = △ACE, and △CEY = 1 acre and △ACE = 3 acres).

The three areas already accounted for total 7 acres, so the quadrilateral BYED is 5 acres.

Both △ABC and △CBD are 6 acres; the remaining plots up to 11 acres can be found by subtracting the parts mentioned above from the whole.

360. Let Andy begin with B blue socks and G gray socks. Then:

$$\frac{B}{B + G} \times \frac{B - 1}{B + G - 1} + \frac{G}{B + G} \times \frac{G - 1}{B + G - 1} = \frac{1}{2}$$

From which $B^2 + G^2 - 2BG - B - G = 0$, so $(B - G)^2 = B + G$. Similarly, let Andy end up with B' blue socks and G' gray socks; then $(B' - G')^2 = B' + G'$.

Since $(B' + G') - (B + G) = 2 \times 24$, we then know that $(B' - G')^2 - (B - G)^2 = 48$. The only pairs of perfect squares that differ by 48 are 1, 49; 16, 64; and 121, 169. The first and third of these solutions are inadmissible because they require an odd number of socks. Therefore Andy started with 16 socks and now has 64.

For the record, Andy started with 3 blue pairs and 5 gray pairs (or the other way around), and thanks to his aunt, now has 14 blue pairs and 18 gray pairs (or the other way around).

314. Thomas started with 251 sugar cubes and made a $6 \times 6 \times 6$ cube, a $3 \times 3 \times 3$ cube, and a $2 \times 2 \times 2$ cube. Once the dog ate one sugar cube, Thomas then made two cubes, each $5 \times 5 \times 5$.

373. A triangle measuring 12 by 16 by 20 will just fit inside a triangle measuring 11 by 60 by 61.

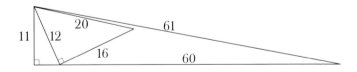

415. $3.16, $1.50, $1.25, and $1.20.
364. 51983.

324. Three planes are needed. The planes set off together and fly one eighth of the way around the world. One then tops the other two up with fuel before returning to base. The other two planes continue until they are a quarter of the way around the world, then one tops up the other with fuel and returns to base. The remaining plane then flies solo until it is three quarters of the way around the world when the above maneuvers are carried out in reverse: one plane meets the first plane at the three-quarter point and gives it a quarter tank of gas; then the two planes fly to the seven-eighths point, where they are met by the third plane, who gives them each another quarter tank of gas. All three planes then use their remaining quarter of a tank to return to base.

377. The integers from 1 to 27 total 378, and in a $3 \times 3 \times 3$ magic cube will appear as nine rows (or columns or pillars). The common sum for this magic cube must therefore be $378 \div 9 = 42$.

Each cell of the top layer of the cube connects to a cell on the bottom layer of the cube via the cell at the center of the cube. These nine lines total $9 \times 42 = 378$. The top layer and bottom layer of the cube both comprise three rows, so between them total $6 \times 42 = 252$. The center cell of the magic cube described in the question must always therefore be $(378 - 252) \div 9 = 14$.

One such magic cube is shown below.

27	11	4
5	25	12
10	6	26

13	9	20
21	14	7
8	19	15

2	22	18
16	3	23
24	17	1

413. There are five ways that Wink can win the best of nine games: 5–0, 5–1, 5–2, 5–3, or 5–4. The respective probabilities of these are: $(1/3)^5$, $(1/3)^5 \times 2/3 \times 5$, $(1/3)^5 \times (2/3)^2 \times 15$, $(1/3)^5 \times (2/3)^3 \times 35$, and $(1/3)^5 \times (2/3)^4 \times 70$. These total 14.5%.

For Wink to win from being down 3–2, he must win three games in a row, or three out of the next four. The probability of this is $(1/3)^3 + (1/3)^3 \times 2/3 \times 3 = 11.1\%$.

Wink should not accept Tiddle's offer. Tiddle could just as well have said, "In nine games, I expect to win 6–3; shall we call it 5–3?" By not accepting Tiddle's offer, Wink risks losing by 5–0 or 5–1, but also leaves more room for luck to work in his favor.

362. Label the five inventors N, O, P, Q, and R, and label their respective inventions as n, o, p, q, and r, where "r" represents the robot. The table below shows the 13 crossings required.

First bank	Boat		Second bank
NOPQR, nopqr			—
NOPQR, pq	nor	⟶	nor
NOPQR, pqr	⟵	r	no
NOPQR, q	pr	⟶	nopr
NOPQR, qr	⟵	r	nop
QR, qr	NOP	⟶	NOP, nop
NQR, nqr	⟵	Nn	OP, op
NQ, nq	Rr	⟶	OPR, opr
NOQ, noq	⟵	Oo	PR, pr
noq	NOQ	⟶	NOPQR, pr
noqr	⟵	r	NOPQR, p
q	nor	⟶	NOPQR, nopr
qr	⟵	r	NOPQR, nop
—	qr	⟶	NOPQR, nopqr

378. Since the ten digits add up to 45, and each is counted twice when the sums are formed, the average sum must be $2 \times 45 \div 10 = 9$. Clearly every pair cannot add up to 9, so there must be at least two different sums.

If there were only two different sums, then one sum would be under 9 and the other would be over 9. However, consider the circle containing the 9. The numbers in the circles on either side of it must be different, so adding each of them to 9 cannot give the same total. Thus we would have two different sums equal to or greater than the required average of 9, which contradicts the initial assumption. Thus there must be at least three different totals.

The diagram below shows one way in which the ten numbers can be arranged to give just three different totals, in this case 8, 9, and 10.

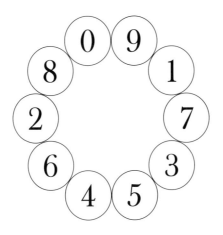

313. Metallica.

342. M, I, and C, spelling "microcosmic."

388. Understudy. The other words contain three consecutive letters of the alphabet; "understudy" has four.

357. The first diagram has one small square in the center; the second diagram has one small square and two large ones.

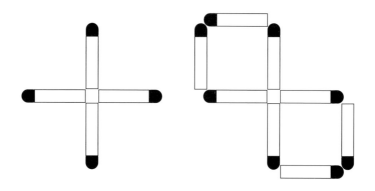

369. $(8 - \sqrt{9})! \times (.9 + \sqrt{.\overline{1}}) = 120 \times .9 + 120 \times .\overline{3} = 108 + 40 = 148$

397. The eight names, from top to bottom, are Nicholas, Jennifer, Geoffrey, Patricia, Benjamin, Samantha, Jonathan, and Rosemary.

348. Breakfast, dinner, tea, supper. The theme is "meals."

412. The question, once the missing vowels (including Y) have been replaced, reads: "What is the lowest whole number that would not be described uniquely if it were written in the same style as this question?" The answer is 8, as "ght" could mean "eight" or "eighty."

327. $2592 = 2^5 \times 9^2$.

380. The divisors of 672 are 1, 2, 3, 4, 6, 7, 8, 12, 14, 16, 21, 24, 28, 32, 42, 48, 56, 84, 96, 112, 168, 224, 336, and 672, which total 2,016, or 3×672.

306. The first sticker Hayley buys will, naturally, not duplicate another sticker she already owns. Buying a second sticker she doesn't already own (we'll call that a "useful sticker" for convenience) will require an average of 250/249 purchases. This is the sum of:

$$1 \times \frac{249}{250} + 2 \times \frac{1}{250} \times \frac{249}{250} + 3 \times \frac{1}{250} \times \frac{1}{250} \times \frac{249}{250} + \ldots$$

The third useful sticker requires an average of 250/248 purchases, and so on. To buy a complete set of 250 stickers this way would therefore cost on average:

$$(1 + \frac{250}{249} + \frac{250}{248} + \frac{250}{247} + \ldots + \frac{250}{2} + 250) \times 20\text{¢} = \$305.03$$

Using a similar formula, the average cost of buying a complete set of 250 stickers by buying stickers one at a time until getting 225 different stickers, and then buying a pack of the remaining 25 stickers would be $114.24 + $12.50 = $126.74. Obviously that's a better option than buying no packs of 25, but it can still be improved upon. A chart of the expected costs of the different options is shown below:

Packs of 25	1	2	3	4	5
Total cost	$126.74	$105.07	$97.47	$95.66	$97.06
Packs of 25	6	7	8	9	10
Total cost	$100.47	$105.29	$111.13	$117.76	$125.00

Hayley should collect 150 individual stickers before ordering four packs of specified stickers if she wants to minimize her costs.

351. The murder was committed by Mrs. Peacock with the candlestick in the conservatory.

401. Indira Gandhi (in DIRA, G and HI).

418. There were 6 + 7 = 13 games where the player that threw first went on to win the game. There were therefore 25 − 13 = 12 games where the player that went first ended up losing the game.

The order of play for the next game changes when a player that went first loses the game. Given that Alvin threw first in the first game and that there were an even number of games (12) where the player that threw first lost the game, it follows that Alvin would have thrown first had there been a 26th game. Alvin must therefore have won the 25th game and the tournament.

385.

3	7	6	2	4	5	1
1	34	4	36	5	30	5
4	6	3	5	7	1	2
5	35	7	32	1	28	4
7	2	1	5	3	4	6
6	28	2	25	2	35	3
2	3	5	1	6	4	7

337.

Basket 1	Basket 2
Weight up	Prince down
Queen down	Prince up
Nothing up	Weight down
King down	Weight and Queen up
Nothing up	Weight down
Prince down	Weight up
Nothing up	Weight down
Queen down	Prince up
Weight up	Prince down

368. Let a, b, and c represent the sides of the triangle. We know that $a^2 + b^2 = c^2$ and $ab = 666{,}666 \times 2 = 2^2 \times 3^2 \times 7 \times 11 \times 13 \times 37$.

Either a or b is divisible by 37. Since a and b are interchangeable at this point, let's just say that a is the one divisible by 37, and that $a' = a \div 37$. Since $a \geq 666$, then $a' \geq 18$. Since $b \geq 666$ and $ab = 666{,}666 \times 2$, then $a \leq 2{,}002$ and $a' \leq 54$.

As a and b (and therefore a' and b) do not share a common factor, possible factors of a' are 4, 7, 9, 11, and 13. Since $18 \leq a' \leq 54$, then $a' = 28, 36, 44,$ or 52 and $a = 1{,}036,$ $1{,}332, 1{,}628,$ or $1{,}924$.

By elimination, $a = 1{,}924$, $b = 693$, and c (the hypotenuse) $= 2{,}045$.

316. The distances between the six gas stations are 1, 3, 2, 7, 8, and 10 miles.

399. The capital of Norway is Oslo, which is in the word CzechOSLOvakia.

305.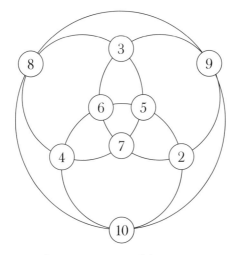

Alternate solutions are possible.

344. In the diagram below, C is the camp, BC is the road across the desert, T is where the traveler begins his journey, and TB is the route due east from the traveler to the road that goes to the camp.

If the direct route TC took 12 units of time to travel, then going from T to C via B would take $5 + {}^{13}/_2 = 11.5$ units of time. The traveler should use the road, then, but where would be the best place to join it?

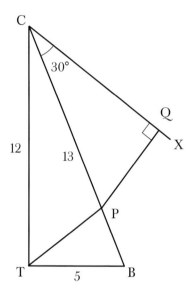

Construct a line CX such that $\angle BCX$ is 30°. Suppose that the traveler goes from T to a random point P on line BC and then, instead of going along the road to C, goes to a point Q on line CX such that $\angle PQC$ is 90°. PQ = ½PC (because the short side of a triangle with angles of 30°, 60°, and 90° is always half the hypotenuse; this can be visualized by imagining an equilateral triangle sliced in half), so the traveler would reach Q at exactly the same time as he would have gotten to C, since it takes twice as long to travel on the desert as on the road.

The traveler's quickest journey to Q would occur when TPQ is a straight line, so he should take the path TP such that ∠TPB = 60°, as shown below.

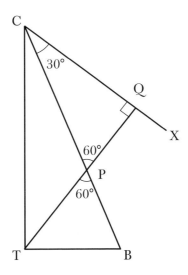

405. The digits a, b, and c are 1, 2, and 7 respectively. $127 = 2^7 - 1$.

321. $12,252,239 = 2^4 \times 3^2 \times 5 \times 7 \times 11 \times 13 \times 17 - 1$

390. The left side of the equation, $[3 \times (300 + n)]^2$, has the factor 3^2 and so is divisible by 9. Therefore the right side of the equation, $898,d04$, must also have 9 as a factor. If a number has a factor of 9, then the sum of its digits is also divisible by 9. Hence d must be 7, from which $n = 16$.

352. Wanda uses a rectangular box measuring 36 by 48 inches, which has a diagonal length of 60 inches.

Also from Puzzlewright Press

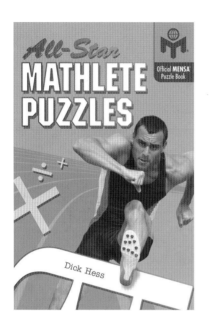

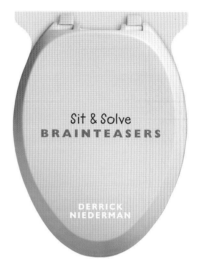

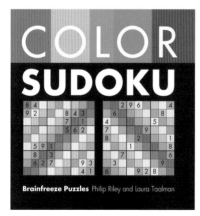

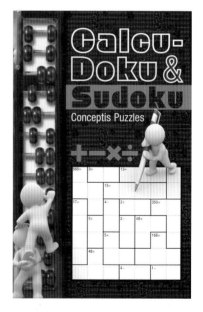